Pocket Guide to

Breastfeeding and Human Lactation

Second Edition

Jan M. Riordan
EdD, ARNP, IBCLC, FAAN
Associate Professor, School of Nursing
Wichita State University

Kathleen G. Auerbach
PhD, IBCLC
University of British Columbia
Vancouver, BC, Canada

D0154657

JONES AND BARTLETT PUBLISHERS
Sudbury, Massachusetts
BOSTON   TORONTO   LONDON   SINGAPORE

World Headquarters
Jones and Bartlett Publishers
40 Tall Pine Drive
Sudbury, MA 01776
978-443-5000
www.jbpub.com
info@jbpub.com

Jones and Bartlett Publishers Canada
2406 Nikanna Road
Mississauga, Ontario
CANADA L5C 2W6

Jones and Bartlett Publishers International
Barb House, Barb Mews
London W6 7PA
UK

ISBN: 0-7637-1469-0

Library of Congress Cataloging-in-Publication Data
Riordan, Jan
  Pocket guide to Breastfeeding and human lactation/Jan M. Riordan,
Kathleen G. Auerbach.–2nd ed.
    p. cm.
  Includes bibliographical references.
  ISBN 0-7637-1469-0
    1. Breast feeding–Handbooks, manuals, etc. 2.
Lactation–Handbooks, manuals, etc.
  [DNLM: 1. Breast Feeding–Handbooks. 2. Lactation–Handbooks.
WS 39 R585p 2001] I. Title: Breastfeeding and human lactation.
II. Auerbach, Kathleen G. III. Title.
  RJ216 .R548 2001
  649'.33–dc 21

                                    00-042425

Production Credits
Acquisitions Editor: John Danielowich
Production Editor: Rebecca S. Marks
Editorial/Production Assistant: Christine Tridente
Director of Manufacturing and Inventory Control: Therese Bräuer
Marketing Manager: Lynn Protasowicki
Cover Design: AnnMarie Lemoine
Design and Composition: Carlisle Communications, Ltd.
Cover Illustration: Marcia Smith
Printing and Binding: Courier Westford
Cover printing: Courier Westford

Printed in the United States of America
03 02 01 00   10 9 8 7 6 5 4 3 2 1

CONTENTS

iv

APPENDICES

Breast, Assessment

Breasts come in all sizes and shapes (see color plates 1–21 in Auerbach and Riordan, *Clinical Lactation: A visual guide,* 1999).

The first step in physical assessment is a thorough handwashing. Next, explain to the client what you are planning to do and ask her permission to do so. Help the client remove all of her upper clothing. With the client in a sitting position, place a clean sheet or light blanket around her shoulders. As you move through the assessment, address these areas:

Inspection

General breast: Are the breasts small, medium, large?
   During pregnancy, breasts normally enlarge so this is an important (even critical) question to ask if the woman is pregnant. Breasts come in many variations of shapes and sizes. In most cases, and despite variations in size and shape, the breasts provide adequate breastmilk for the baby's needs. While size is not important per se, marked differences between one breast and the other should be noted, as this finding may be associated with milk production problems (see Breast, Hypoplasia).

Nipple and areola: The size of the nipple is not important except when it is very small or very large. This nipple size can become a breastfeeding problem if there is a disparity between the nipple size and the size of the baby. For example, women with very large nipples will need extra help in putting a preterm or small neonate to breast.

Skin: Note any marks or unusual areas on the skin. Are there any surgical scars? Red areas? Lesions? Surgical scars, especially at or near the areolar margin may result in reduced sensation and possible trauma to the ducts. A lateral incision in the vicinity of the cutaneous branch of the fourth intercostal nerve (left breast, 5 o'clock position; right breast, 7 o'clock position) from augmentation or reduction surgery may have caused severed innervation of the nipple and areola. Surgery on the breast, especially if it involves an incision at the areolar margin, is likely to interfere at least to some degree with milk production. Some women will not volunteer information that they have had breast surgery. In some cases, the surgeon's skill was such that scarring is extremely difficult to identify. The wise practitioner will include a question such as, "Have you ever had any surgery to your breast or chest area for any reason?" in order to rule out such a history as a cause of breastfeeding difficulties.

Check for skin tags—near or around the nipple, skin tags can interfere with feedings. If the mother is lactating, note any area of redness that might suggest a plugged duct or mastitis.

Palpation

Nipple protractibility: Assess nipple size and eversion or inversion of the nipple. Does the nipple look everted, flat, inverted? Gently compress the area behind the nipple to see if the nipple tissue everts. If the nipple is clearly inverted, record this finding. The aim of the plan of care is to reduce any effect of nipple inversion on breastfeeding. Prenatal teaching should begin early and include information about how the patient can become familiar with her breasts and their reactivity to various forms of stimulation. When the nipple is compressed using the pinch test, it responds in one of the ways identified in Figure 2. This response may reflect degree of function.

Palpation of breasts: After assessing nipple protractibility, gently palpate the remaining breast tissue as you would in a self-breast exam. Are there any thick or lumpy areas? Ask the mother to raise one arm at a time and palpate the area above the breast into her axilla for possible supernumerary breast tissue. Look for any small pigmented spots that may suggest a tiny supernumerary areola.

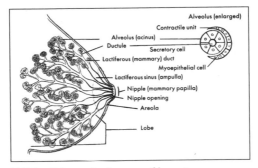

FIG 1   Schematic diagram of breast.

4

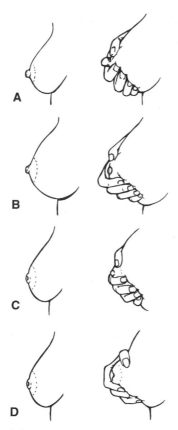

FIG 2   A - D Nipple Function
A. Protracting normal nipple. B. Moderate to
severe retraction. C. Inverted-appearing nipple,
which, when compressed using pinch test, will
either invert farther inward or will protract
forward (upper right). D. True inversion; nipple
inverts further (lower right).

Breast, Creams and Gels

General information (research-based) on treatment for sore nipples:

- Applying breastmilk or warm water on the nipple area is as effective as commercial creams or ointments for treating sore nipples (Lavergne 1997).
- USP Modified Lanolin that promotes moist wound healing or keeps tissue soft is somewhat effective for sore nipples.
- Wearing breast shells and applying lanolin is effective treatment for sore nipples (Brent et al. 1998).
- Apply the ointment/cream sparingly after the feeding. Creams that must be washed off should not be used, for such action defeats the purpose of using the cream and exacerbates the tenderness.

COMMERCIAL PRODUCTS USED FOR NIPPLE SORENESS

NAME	DESCRIPTION/INGREDIENTS	COMMENTS
A&D Ointment	Ointment in tube. Contains anhydrous lanolin, petrolatum, fragrance, mineral oil, fish liver oil, and chaolecalciferol.	There are no vitamins in this ointment.
Bag Balm	Stiff yellow ointment. Contains petrolatum, lanolin, 8-hydroxyquinoline sulfate, sanitas, and water.	A fungistat and bactericide for farm use. *Not for internal use* since 1969, for causing cancer in laboratory animals.
Hydrogel occlusive wound dressing (Elasto-gel, ClearSite)	Glycerin-based hydrogel. Absorbent, nonadhesive, bacteriostatic, and fungistatic. Dressing 1/8-in thick with soothing, cooling properties for pain relief.	Wound dressings sealed in sterile package. Can be purchased in pharmacy area. $5 for package of 4. Do not appear to be effective in preventing and treating sore nipples in women who breastfeed (Brent et al. 1998).

Product	Composition	Comments
Massé Cream	Glyceryl stearate, glycerin, cetyl alcohol, stearate, stearic acid, polysorbate 60, propylparaben, methylparaben, potassium hydroxide.	Instructions advise to cleanse the breasts before and after each nursing with a clean cloth and water. Not recommended.
USP Modified Lanolin (Lansinoh, Purelan, Marcalan)	100% anhydrous, modified lanolin.	Hypoallergenic. Estimated to contain under 1.5 ppm of combined impurities. Used in moist healing.
USP Lanolin (Merck "Lanum")	Tube or cream. Contains hydrous lanolin.	Highly allergenic wool derivative. Analysis revealed all contained organophosphorous pesticide residue including diazinon.
Vaseline Petroleum Jelly	Gel in a jar. Contains white petrolatum.	Not recommended for sore nipples.
Vitamin E (generic)	Vitamin capsules, oil, gelatin, or cream. Contains Vitamin E in suspension. Capsules = 400 IU each.	US recommended RDA for Vitamin E in infants is 5 IU/day. Effect of increased serum concentrations of Vitamin E is unknown.

Breast, Eczema, Impetigo, Psoriasis

General information:

Dermatitis with rash, itching, and burning. Breast/nipple is dark pink to red. Skin is flaky and dry. Differentiate between eczema, impetigo, and psoriasis (see color plates 32, 33, 34, 37, 38 in *Clinical lactation: A visual guide*).

Bacterial infection (impetigo): Complaints of nipple pain with cracks, fissures, ulcers, or exudate. Of these women, there is a 64% chance of having a positive bacterial skin culture.

Obtain a nipple culture from an unwashed cracked nipple before breastfeeding, using a cotton-tipped culturette.

Medical treatment options for impetigo:

- Antibacterial topical ointment to affected area.
- Oral antibiotic therapy: penicillinase resistant (dicloxacillin, cephalosporin, erythromycin).

Guidelines for Care

- If identified, remove the causative irritant.
- Apply cool, wet compresses to the affected area.
- Wear loose-fitting clothing and all-cotton bras.
- Wear breast shells with multiple air holes for 6–8 hrs/day. Keep the breasts exposed to air as much as possible.
- Expose breasts to filtered sunlight 2× daily for 15–20 minutes.
- Apply antibacterial cream (Bacitracin, Bactroban)
- Apply 0.5% hydrocortisone cream (available OTC). In some cases, an anti-

inflammatory cream or other emollient may be helpful.[1]

Continue breastfeeding; if problem persists, seek assessment from skilled practitioner familiar with the condition.

[1]Caution: If thrush is also present, a steroid cream may worsen the condition.

Breast, Expression by Hand

Hand expression of breastmilk is a time-honored skill. No special equipment is needed; a woman's hands are always available and the technique costs nothing. Women who are experienced in hand expression of breastmilk claim they can obtain more milk more quickly than with a breast pump.

Guidelines for Hand Expression
(takes about 20–30 minutes)

A. Wash hands and collection container. Apply a warm, moist towel or take a warm shower to enhance flow. Gently massage the breast starting at the top, pressing firmly into the chest wall. Use gentle pressure in a circular motion and move around the breast.

B. Position the thumb and first two fingers about 1 to 1 1/2 inches behind the nipple and press into the chest.

C. Roll the thumb and fingers forward. This rolling motion compresses and empties the milk sinuses without damaging the sensitive breast tissue. Repeat to drain all the milk ducts.

D. Rotate the thumb and finger position to compress all milk ducts on both breasts. Express each breast until the flow of milk slows or stops.

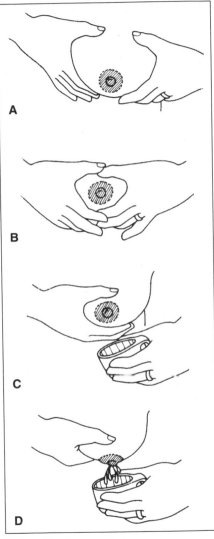

FIG 3   Hand expression.

Breast, Hypoplasia

A rare condition associated with delayed and inadequate milk supply and characterized by 1) marked asymmetry of the breasts and/or nipples and/or areolae, 2) a space between the breasts greater than one inch (2.5 cm), 3) slow weight gain in the infant unless supplemented, 4) infant not satiated following vigorous, apparently effective suckling. The mother may also report few breast changes during pregnancy.

Assess for hypoplasia first by visual observation of both breasts. (See color plates 85, 86, 87, 88, and 90 in *Clinical lactation: A visual guide*). Visualize both breasts simultaneously. A wide space between the breasts indicates the likelihood of substantially delayed or inadequate milk production.

Guidelines for Care

Supplementation, preferably at the breast, is needed. Supplementation, preferably by a method that keeps the baby on the breast, may be necessary during the interim period.

Encourage the mother to meet with a skilled lactation consultant so that the mother and baby can be followed carefully and the baby's nutritional needs are met while the mother is developing a milk supply or until it is determined that she may need to supplement long-term.

Breast, Lump

General information:

Breast lumps in lactating women are most often a galactocele or milk-filled lacteal cyst. If it does not resolve spontaneously, a thorough medical assessment should be made to determine the type of blockage and possible pathology, and to rule out breast cancer. Although breast cancer is rare in pregnant and/or breastfeeding women, a lump in the breast should never be ignored.

- Monitor for any changes in the size of the lump.
- Aspirate to determine if the lump is fluid-filled or if it appears to be a cystic mass.
- Refer the mother to a medical specialist, preferably an experienced surgeon.
- Evaluate the nature of a solid breast mass by performing ultrasound and, if indicated, a biopsy.
- Continue breastfeeding. Continuing feeding from the affected breast following biopsy is possible as long as the incision site is not close to the nipple and that the baby's mouth does not cause discomfort.

Breast, Mammaplasty (Reduction and Augmentation)

The mother's ability to breastfeed following mammaplasty depends on the type of surgery, specific technique used, whether neural pathways were severed, and the amount of tissue removed. Generally, breastfeeding is possible following augmentation surgery. Milk production following reduction surgery may be inadequate to sustain exclusive breastfeeding and satisfactory infant growth. The probability of adequate milk production increases if the surgeon attempts to leave nerve pathways, milk ducts, and the blood supply intact. Breastfeeding is more likely if the pedicle technique (in which the nipple remains attached to the breast while surrounding tissue is removed) is used; adequate milk transfer is rarely possible with the free nipple technique, in which the nipple is removed and then repositioned on the reshaped/resculpted breast. (See color plates 74, 75, 76, 77, 78, and 79 in *Clinical lactation: A visual guide*.)

Guidelines for Care

- Assess the extent and type of surgery. If incision scars are not periareolar, the mother is more likely to be able to sustain adequate breastfeeding without supplementation.
- Counsel the mother that breastfeeding is possible and encourage her to initiate breastfeeding. Ability to produce milk among these women varies widely and cannot be predicted. Each case must be treated individually.
- Carefully monitor the mother for signs of milk ejection and production. Assess infant for adequate hydration and growth.

- Early adequacy may not predict later adequacy of milk production as the baby's need for larger volumes increases. Continued follow-up is necessary to assure adequate milk transfer in order to sustain normal infant growth.
- Offer techniques for supplementation if the infant needs additional nutrition, such as cup feeding and feeding tube systems (see page 28).

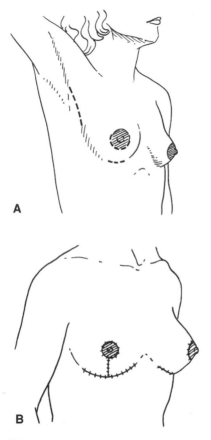

FIG 4   A. Augmentation surgery: Incision is
made through the armpit, underneath the breast,
or under the areola.
B. Reduction surgery: Postoperative appearance.

Breast, Pain

General information:

Intermittent pain and soreness in breast. Pain may be described as "shooting" or "deep," often occurring during and after feedings.

ASSESS FOR:	GUIDELINES FOR CARE
Bra fit	Suggest comfortable, supportive bra without underwires
Breast lumps	See pp. 13
Candida, thrush	See pp. 31
Mastitis	See pp. 82
Milk ejection (letdown)	See Milk ejection
Underlying muscle pain from upper body exertion	Discomfort usually resolves spontaneously; suggest over the counter (OTC) pain med such as ibuprofen

Breast, Preference

General information:

Occasionally, a baby will prefer to nurse from one breast only or from one breast more consistently than the other.

Assess for possible causes:
- Mother's skill in positioning the baby on each breast. The mother's dominant side can contribute to her feeling more comfortable holding the baby to one breast but not the other.
- Unilateral paresis, weakness, or other physical factors affect how the mother holds the baby to the breast.
- Baby's position *in utero,* particularly during the last month of the pregnancy. This position preference usually fades on its own after several days or a week.
- Otitis media, facial paralysis, swelling, and tenderness from an assisted forceps birth, broken clavicle.

Guidelines for Care

- Instruct the mother in how to bring the baby to breast with a minimum of positioning changes, starting on the side the baby accepts and then moving him or her to the less-preferred side.
- Assist the mother to position the baby on both breasts without putting undo pressure on the broken clavicle (if this is present).
- Offer the unpreferred breast when baby is not fully awake.
- Assure the mother that in most cases, such breast preference is transient.
- If the preference persists and the baby continues to gain weight well, reassure the mother that feeding from one breast is

adequate. If she has concerns about breast asymmetry stemming from breastfeeding on only one side, discuss ways in which she can alter her clothing to minimize the differences in breast size during the breastfeeding course.

Breast, Pumps

General information:

Many kinds of breast pumps are available. The best pump to use in any given situation will depend on the mother's reason for needing a pump and the costs involved in its use. Battery-operated or manual pumps are best for short-term use. Fully automated electric pumps are best for long-term use, especially for mothers of hospitalized preterm or ill infants. A certified lactation consultant (IBCLC) can recommend accessible and appropriate pumps.

Types of Pumps:

Manual: Pressure is created by hand squeeze action. Fatigue is a drawback. For short-term use only.

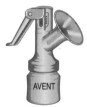

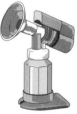

FIG 5-A   Avent Pump.

FIG 5-B   Medela mini-electric battery-operated pump.

Do not use bicycle horn pumps!   Their design is faulty, and they cannot be cleaned adequately to avoid contamination of the breastmilk obtained.

FIG 5-C   Bicycle horn pump.

Cylinder: Easy to use and relatively inexpensive. Price range is $12–$30. Two concentric cylinders fit together and are joined with a gasket seal. As the outer cylinder is pulled outward, a suction is created. Milk collects in the outer cylinder. As the outer cylinder fills, the pressure increases. In some cases, such cylinder models must be emptied several times to avoid overfilling and spillage.

FIG 5-D Straight-head pump.

FIG 5-E Angled-head cylinder pump.

Battery-operated: Primary advantage is portability. Major disadvantage is the need for batteries. Best are those with rechargeable batteries, which do not require frequent replacement. Prices range from $35 to $95.

FIG 5-F Gentle Expressions Pump.

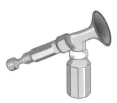

FIG 5-G Medela Mini-electric pump.

Electric (Semiautomated): Suction is created when the user alternately creates and releases pressure. Purchase cost is about $100. Not always sufficient for sustained long-term pumping or if the mother has not yet established an adequate milk supply.

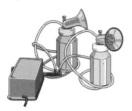

FIG 5-H   Nurture III semiautomatic pump. (Bailey Medical Engineering)

Electric (Fully automated):   Has alternating suction which attempts to imitate the baby feeding at the breast. A dual hookup system where the mother can pump both breasts simultaneously reduces overall pumping time. Daily charges are approximately $1–$4; starter kits that contain tubing and bottles cost about $25–$55. Purchase cost about $1,200. Use if pumping will last longer than 1–2 months. Most women only rent these pumps if they anticipate long-term use for more than one child.

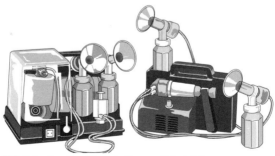

FIG 5-I   Lactina Electric Pumps (Medela).

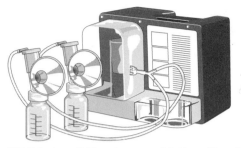

FIG 5-J   Lact-E Electric pump. (Hollister/Ameda-Egnell)

Suggestions for using a mechanical breast pump:
· Wash all parts that touch the mother's skin
  or her milk, rinsing first in cold water, and
  then washing well in hot soapy water,
  rinsing in hot water, and allowing to air dry.
· Check the manufacturers' instructions
  regarding the safety of washing in
  mechanical dishwashers.
· Store milk in containers holding about the
  amount the baby is expected to take in a
  given feeding.
· Store small amounts of milk for "desserts"
  or "between-meal snacks" that will keep the
  baby satisfied.
· Store raw unrefrigerated milk for several
  hours (capped, out of the sun or other heat
  source).
· Keep milk clean during transportation from
  the pumping site to the home or where the
  baby is cared for. Refrigerate or freeze the
  milk immediately after arriving home.
· Store milk in the back of the refrigerator or
  freezer. (Milk stored on the door varies in
  temperature and is more likely to sour.)
· Use the oldest milk first.

- Use refrigerated milk within 4–8 days.
- Use frozen milk within two weeks unless deep frozen at 0°F. Older milk will be usable, but it may have "off-odors"or taste. The baby may refuse to take it.
- Use milk within 6 months if deep frozen.

Guidelines for Pumping

Advise mother to:

- Wash her hands thoroughly with soap and water. Prepare a clean container in which to store her milk.
- Take deep breaths to relax; drink juice or water before and during pumping.
- Allow sufficient time for pumping. Duration of 10–15 minutes with an electric pump is usually adequate; 10–20 minutes may be needed with manual or battery-operated pump. Double pumping with a dual setup electric or two battery-operated pumps is usually complete within 7–15 minutes.
- Use only as much suction as is needed to maintain milk flow.
- Massage the breasts during pumping to increase intramammary pressure and flow when pumping one breast at a time.
- Stop pumping when milk flow is minimal or has ceased.

Breast, Refusal

General information:

Occasionally, a baby will be reluctant to, or refuse to, accept one or both breasts. Assess how the mother is positioning and holding the baby at breast. Pushing the baby's face into the breast may result in the baby's refusal to nurse and a change in how the baby roots when put to breast.

Assess for a possible broken clavicle; in some cases, infant discomfort when lying on the affected side may appear as unilateral breast refusal.

Guidelines for Care

- Instruct the mother in how to bring the baby to breast without pressing against the back of the baby's head.
- Assist the mother to position the baby on both breasts without putting undo pressure on the broken clavicle (if this is present).
- If refusal is unilateral, use the opposite breast first and then slide baby into position on the other breast with minimal positioning changes.
- If refusal is bilateral, offer breast when baby is not fully awake.
- If refusal becomes consistent, consider a period of feeding the baby expressed human milk to extinguish the aversive response. Gentle, patient encouragement is especially important here.
- Assure the mother that the baby is not rejecting her or her milk, only a position that he or she has learned to fear.

Breast, Self-Examination*

Breast self-examination should be encouraged in all women at least once monthly. Such examination has proven itself a valuable early detection tool of breast changes that may signal growth of tumors, benign or cancerous.

Teach the breastfeeding woman these simple steps to breast self-examination.

1. Stand, nude from the waist up, in front of a mirror, with your arms and hands at your side. Examine the look of your breasts. If you note any change in size or shape, report them to your care provider.
2. Still standing, lean over and note how the breasts hang. If any puckering of the skin is noted, this information should be shared with your care provider.
3. Lie down on a flat surface. Raise one arm over your head. With the other hand, begin palpating your breast tissue, starting under your armpit and working down over the breast until your fingers are below the lowest portion of your breast tissue. Continue this up and down palpation until you no longer feel breast tissue in your cleavage. Repeat with the other breast. If any lumps not previously felt or any change in the size or shape of a previously identified lump is noted, this information should be shared with your care provider.

*Note: previous instructions in breast self-examination suggested circular palpation around the breast and nipple; however, this technique is more likely to miss a tumor lying just under the nipple. The vertical method is now recommended and is considered more likely to identify changes involving the tissue immediately surrounding and underneath the nipple.

Remember, most lumps are benign; those that are not are more easily removed when discovered early. Most changes in breast lumps are normal; knowing the contours of your breasts (both external and internal) through breast self-examination is a proactive behavior only you can practice! Practice preventive health care by examining your breasts monthly (in the middle of a menstrual cycle if not pregnant).

Breastmilk, Collection and Storage

General information:

How and in what manner breastmilk is stored will depend upon the health status of the infant recipient and such variables as where the mother and baby live and what options are available. Generally, storage and handling recommendations used for sick and premature infants are not used when the infant is full-term, healthy, and cared for at home. Storage guidelines offered here are conservative and may be superceded by protocols and guidelines that provide greater flexibility.

Full-term Infant Storage Guidelines in the Hospital

In general, hospital guidelines must take into account the greater likelihood that the recipient will be ill, may be receiving milk from a mother other than his or her own, and that resistant organisms are more likely to exist in the hospital environment.

- Encourage mothers to express their milk on site after washing their hands thoroughly, paying particular attention to their nails. There is no need to wash the breasts.
- Accept milk that is expressed elsewhere if it is transported on ice or fully frozen on arrival in the unit.
- Label all milk with the baby's name, the mother's name, and the date and time of its expression.
- Prepare for use only the amount of milk that is likely to be used by the baby. This will reduce unnecessarily wasting "liquid gold."
- Encourage the mother to bring in her milk in aliquots that closely match what the baby is being given.

- Provide the mother with ample milk storage containers.
- Keep all milk frozen until used.

Use milk in the following order:
1. Fresh raw milk expressed within one hour prior to its use. If the mother expresses longer than 1 hour in advance of the baby's next feeding, refrigerate the extra milk for the baby's next feeding.
2. Refrigerated milk less than 48 hours old (if milk is to be used after more than 48 hours, freeze it).
3. Frozen milk (oldest first).

Low Birth Weight Infant Storage Guidelines for NICU

- Whenever possible, breastmilk should be fed fresh in order to retain its maximum infection-fighting properties.
- Keep fresh, unrefrigerated milk at room temperature for up to 2 hours or refrigerate it for up to 48 hours. Discard any refrigerated milk unused after 48 hours.
- Store frozen milk at $< -20°C$ until thawed for infant feeding. After thawing, store milk in the refrigerator for up to 24 hours. Discard any thawed milk unused after 24 hours.

Storage Guidelines in the Home

Suggestions for hand expressing:
- Wash hands well, paying particular attention to the nails, before expressing milk.
- Express milk into a clean container; DO NOT touch the inside of the container when capping same.

Heating Guidelines

- *Defrosting should occur within about 15 minutes* to minimize a reduction in immunological properties. Avoid slow/gradual thawing in the refrigerator, at room temperature, or in a pan of lukewarm water.

- *Defrost frozen milk shortly before use.* Hold the container under cool running water and gradually add warmer water until the milk is thawed and heated to room temperature. Shake the container before testing the temperature.
- *Do not microwave breastmilk.* Such heating destroys vitamin C and other elements in the milk, changes protein composition, markedly increases bacterial growth, and may result in burning the infant's mouth owing to uneven heating of the fluid, even though the container remains cool to the touch.

Candida/Thrush

General information:

Most commonly occurs in the breastfeeding mother and infant following antibiotic treatment. Manifestations include striking, deep pink areas radiating from the nipple area, shiny skin, acute pain during and after breastfeeding; in severe cases, blisters that weep may appear. Mother often complains of severe tenderness and discomfort, especially during and immediately after feedings. (See color plates 40, 41, 42, 43, 44, 45, 46, and 47 in *Clinical lactation: A visual guide.*)

Infant may have a diaper rash with raised, red, angry-looking pustules and/or red scalded-looking buttocks. In severe cases, white spots or patches may be observed in the baby's mouth; baby may appear to be in pain and refuse to suckle or act as if he or she is attempting to scratch the upper palate with the tongue. (See color plates 102, 103, and 104 in *Clinical lactation: A visual guide.*)

Guidelines for Care

- Apply an antifungal topical cream or lotion to nipples and breast after each feeding, and swab the infant's mouth, tongue, and gums after each feeding.
- Suggest that the mother briefly apply ice to her nipples before feeding to reduce pain.
- Ointments and creams are not absorbed through the mucous membranes, so it is not necessary to remove all the ointment before the baby breastfeeds.
- *Treat entire family:* Boil pacifiers, rubber teats, teethers, toys, etc. Use disposable breast pads. In chronic cases, suspect an asymptomatic carrier, often the father. Refer to physician for assessment and treatment of the father for possible candida. Avoid family bathing together.

MEDICATIONS

Drug Name	Preparations	Dosage and Comments
Clotrimazole (Gyne-lotrimin, Mycelex, Lotrimin)	Creams, solutions, vaginal cream Tablet: 100 mg/day for 7 days or 200 mg/day for 3 days.	Apply skin cream twice a day. Potential for minimally elevated liver enzymes.
Clotrimazole and betamethasone (Lotrisone)	Cream to nipples	Combination antifungal and corticosteroid. Helpful for severe nipple pain.
Gentian violet	Adults and children: Topical 0.5%, 1% solution	Infant: 2–3 times over several days. Use diluted 0.5% solution. One-time treatment only.
Fluconazole (Diflucan)	Mother: tablet 200–400 mg stat followed by 100–200 mg daily for at least 2 weeks. Infant: 6 mg/kg stat followed by 3 mg/kg/day	Cleared for pediatric use. Infant receives 1% of maternal dose and <5% of pediatric dose. Preferred over ketoconazole for oral and vaginal candidiasis.

Miconazole (Monistat)	Creams, lotions, vaginal cream and suppositories	Skin cream or lotion: apply 3–4 times/day; vaginal cream or suppository: 100 mg/day for 7 days. Commonly used in pediatric patients <1 year old.
Nystatin and triamcinolone (Mycolog II)	Cream	Combination antifungal and corticosteroid. Helpful for severe nipple pain.
Nystatin	Suspensions, cream, powders, ointment, and vaginal suppositories *Mother:* 1,500,000 U–2,400,000 U/day divided into 3–4 doses *Infant:* 400,000–800,000 U/day, divided into 3–4 doses	Continue therapy at least 2 days after symptoms disappear. *Mother:* Topical cream: apply 2 times/day to nipple area after breastfeeding. Wait 10 minutes before replacing bra. *Infant:* Swab mixed suspension in infant's mouth after feedings with cotton-tipped applicator. Ointment to infant's buttocks after each diapering.

Cesarean Birth

General information:

The woman who has a cesarean birth is also a postoperative patient. If the cesarean birth was unplanned, it may represent a disappointment for the mother; as a result, breastfeeding often takes on special importance.

Guidelines for Care

- Encourage breastfeeding as soon as possible after birth. Early and frequent feeds are as important for these mothers as for those who give birth vaginally.
- Generally, single doses or limited use of narcotics postpartum to relieve maternal pain will not interfere with breastfeeding.
- Use pillows to place the infant in a football (clutch) position so that mother's incisional area is protected while sitting in a chair to breastfeed. Attempting to sit in bed rarely is as comfortable for the mother as using a high-backed chair with low arms and positioning so that her feet are on the floor or pressed against a footrest or stool.
- Place the mother in a flat side-lying position (early postpartum) for feedings if spinal anesthesia was used.

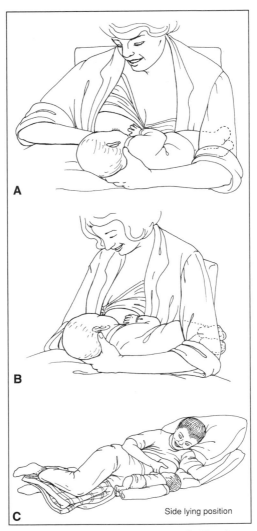

Side lying position

FIG 6   A. Modified clutch position. B. Clutch
hold. C. Side-lying position.

Chickenpox (Varicella Zoster, Virus)

General information:

The infectious period can begin 1–5 days before eruption of vesicles. Lesions begin on neck or trunk and spread to the face, scalp, mucous membrane, and extremities.

Most mothers and hospital personnel have had chickenpox and are not at risk. When a mother develops chickenpox several days before the baby's birth, the infant is at risk because maternal antibodies that confer immunity to the neonate have not yet been produced.

Guidelines for Care

- If the mother is exposed and has already had chickenpox, breastfeeding will confer antibodies to the infant. Interrupting breastfeeding is not necessary.
- If the mother has not had chickenpox, she and her infant should receive the varicella vaccine if they have been exposed.
- If the mother develops chickenpox several days before she delivers her baby:
  - Mother and infant should be isolated separately if the neonate does not develop lesions. Only about 50% of infants exposed will develop the disease.
  - Express the breastmilk if baby is housed elsewhere.
  - If the infant has lesions, isolate the baby with the mother; breastfeeding may occur uninterrupted.

Contraception

General information:

Frequency and length of feedings are closely related to duration of anovulation and amenorrhea. Women who are exclusively breastfeeding will have about 98 percent protection for the first several months.

The 6/60 rule Generally, if feedings occur at least six times per day or at least 60 minutes per day, and night feedings are still occurring, ovulation is unlikely to occur.

FERTILITY CONTROL CHOICES FOR BREASTFEEDING WOMEN

METHODS	WHEN TO START	EFFECT ON MILK PRODUCTION
Barrier methods Condom Cervical cap or diaphragm	Anytime after it is safe to have intercourse postpartum	No effect
Depo-Provera (progestin-only)	Wait until 6 weeks postpartum*	May enhance milk supply
Intrauterine device (IUD)	Wait until 6 weeks postpartum	No effect
Lactational Amenorrhea Method (LAM)	Immediately	Exclusive breastfeeding increases likelihood of abundant milk supply
Natural Family Planning (abstinence or barrier method through 4-day fertile period)	Anytime after it is safe to have intercourse postpartum	No effect

Norplant (progestin-only)	Wait until 6 weeks postpartum*	No effect on milk supply but has other side effects
Oral contraceptives (progestin-only) Micronor (norethindrone) Ovrette (norgestrel)	Wait until 6 weeks postpartum*	In most cases does not affect milk supply
Oral contraceptives COCs (combined estrogen and progestin) Lo/ovral, Norethin	Contraindicated; do not give to lactating women	Substantial reduction of breastmilk supply
Withdrawal	Anytime after it is safe to have intercourse postpartum	No effect

*WHO, 1998

Cup Feeding

When supplements are needed, cup feeding allows an infant to be fed without the risk of developing nipple confusion and preference for rubber nipples. A wide variety of small cups work well, including medicine cups, plastic specimen cups, and shot glasses.

Guidelines

- Wash your hands thoroughly before cup feeding.
- Pour the desired amount of supplement (breastmilk or formula) into a small medicine cup or cup especially designed for infant feeding.
- Place the infant in an upright position, support the head, and lean the baby forward slightly.
- Lightly touch the cup just below the infant's lower lip. As the infant opens his mouth and begins a lapping action, tip the cup slightly until the milk touches the lower lip (DO NOT pour the milk into the infant's mouth).
- The infant should lap up or sip the milk as it touches his lip. Most infants begin cup feeding with a lapping action; later, they will sip from the cup, often bringing their hands around the cup when it is brought to their mouths and smelling the contents of the container.
- If the infant coughs or chokes, stop and lean the infant forward to allow him to clear his throat.

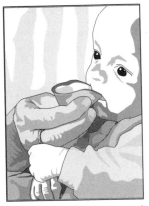

FIG 7　Soft flexible cup for feeding infant
(Maternal Concepts).

Cytomegalovirus (CMV)

General information:

CMV is common; 50–80% of the population have CMV antibodies in their blood. The organism can be found in saliva, urine, and breastmilk. The fetus may be infected *in utero*. The most serious congenital problems occur in infants born to mothers who have primary CMV during pregnancy.

Breastfeeding is an important means of conveying passive immunity to CMV in infants. Breastfed children, who are thus immunized, are protected later in life from symptomatic infection and from primary infection during pregnancy.

Guidelines for Care

Full-term Infant: Encourage breastfeeding for full-term infants if mother was already seropositive during pregnancy. Consumption of infected breastmilk generally leads to CMV infection and thus seroconversion of infants without adverse sequelae.

Preterm Infant: Carefully weigh the risk factors of giving milk from a mother with CMV infection to a premature infant, especially if he or she is seronegative. Defer to neonatologist for evaluation and decision.

Depression, Postpartum

General information:

About 70–80% of women experience a transient depression following birth. The "blues" is usually temporary and occurs within the first week or two. About 20% of postpartum women will experience moderate depression following childbirth. Postpartum psychosis is rare. The onset of psychosis usually occurs within a few days to two weeks after delivery. Symptoms peak at about six weeks postpartum and may be triggered or exacerbated by separation of mother and baby.

Postpartum "blues": tearfulness, mood swings. Is more common in women having their first child, particularly if the mother and baby have been separated. This condition usually disappears after two weeks.

Clinical depression: Sleep disturbances, feelings of insecurity and worthlessness; isolation; lack of supportive relationships.

Psychosis: Insomnia, irrational ideas, feelings of failure, hallucination, self-destructive thoughts.

Guidelines for Care

- Refer to follow-up care with a nurse therapist, psychologist, or psychiatrist.
- Women with postpartum psychosis may need to be hospitalized. Treatment with medication is mandatory.
- The SSRI family are drugs of choice for breastfeeding women experiencing postpartum depression, as they are compatible with breastfeeding and usually work faster than the tricyclics. See table for Drugs Used for Postpartum Depression.

DRUGS USED FOR POSTPARTUM DEPRESSION

Drug Name	Daily Oral Dosage (MG)	Use in Breastfeeding Mother and Safety Level
Serotonin selective reuptake inhibitors (SSRI)		
Citalopram (Celexa)	20	Infants receive 0.4% of the weight-adjusted maternal dose. No untoward effects were reported in breastfed infants.
Fluoxetine (Prozac)	10–40	Infants receive 5–9% of maternal dose. Case reports of infant colic and fussiness. Not recommended for breastfeeding.
Paroxetine (Paxil)	20–50	Minimal levels in breastmilk. Relatively short half-life.
Sertaline (Zoloft)	50–150	No adverse effects reported, and, in almost all cases, no drug detectable in plasma compartment of the infant.
Venlafaxine (Effexor)	75–300	Mean total infant dose was 7.6% of the maternal weight-adjusted dose. No acute adverse effects observed.

Tricyclics

Amitriptyline (Elavil)	50–300	Safe. No effects on infants reported. No apparent accumulation in nursing infant.
Desipramine (Norpramin)	50–300	Relatively safe.
Imipramine (Tofranil)	50–300	Relatively safe. Infant would receive approx. 0.04 mg/kg/day.
Nortriptyline (Pamelor)	25–100	Safe. Not detected in serum of infant.

MAO Inhibitors

Phenelzine (Nardil)	15–90	Contraindicated. Inhibits lactation.
Tranylcypromine (Parnate)	10–30	Use with caution.

(continued)

45

Phenothiazines

Chlorpromazine (Thorazine)	30–1000	Relatively safe if average dosage; one report of infant drowsiness with high dosage. May increase mother's milk supply.
Mesoridazine (Serentil)	100–400	Relatively safe.
Perphenazine (Trilafon)	4–6	Safe. Dose passed to child through milk is only 0.1% of that given the mother.
Thioridazine (Mellaril)	150–800	Relatively safe.

Employment, Maternal

General information:

More employers now recognize the health maintaining qualities of breastfeeding. Thus, continuing to breastfeed after returning to work is increasingly common. About half of new mothers return to work when their infants are very young.

Prenatal Planning for Mothers

- Find out about maternity leave options and benefits available at work, and inform the employer of intentions to breastfeed after returning to work.
- Suggest that the mother consider options such as working part-time, flextime, setting up a home office with computer/modem, or bringing infant to work in the early weeks.
- Plan child care arrangements prenatally to avoid less-than-optimal choices postpartum.
- Find a support person who has enjoyed breastfeeding while working and who can be a mentor.
- Identify services for new mothers provided at the work site. These may include breastfeeding or breast pumping facilities, breast pumps available at minimal or no cost to employees, day care facilities at or near the work site, and/or coverage of the cost of using such facilities.

Early Postpartum

- Breastfeed exclusively to establish lactation.
- Wait as long as possible before returning to work if the mother must be separated from her baby. Research shows that the longer the mother is home with her baby in the first four months postpartum, the easier it is to maintain lactation after returning to work.

- Get household help if at all possible.
- Identify a suitable method of expression. If the mother chooses to use a breast pump, a full-size intermittent electric breast pump is the best choice for ease of use and continued adequate milk production.

Returning to Work

- Stockpile breastmilk before returning to work. Breastmilk can be safely kept in the refrigerator or freezer. Assist the mother with appropriate storage options that are available to her.
- Introduce a cup or a bottle no earlier than 7–10 days before returning to work. If the baby is older than two months, a cup is less likely to be refused than a bottle. Someone other than the mother should offer these substituted feedings at a time when the mother will not be available. Avoid sitting in the mother's "favorite" chair for breastfeeding.

At Work, At Home

- Pump two to three times during work hours in the first two weeks or more if mother is not able to breastfeed. The longest pumping should be at mealtime, particularly if that occurs midway in the workday. Usually, more such pumping sessions are needed in the first six months than for later months.
- Breastfeed right after returning home and as often as the baby requests during the evening (if daytime worker). Infants tend to adjust their feedings around their proximity to their mothers.
- Refrigerate milk at work and transport milk home in a small cooler.
- Place photographs of baby at work to view when expressing/pumping milk.

Engorgement, Breast

General information:

Most women experience breast fullness about three to four days after birth. Such fullness accompanies Lactogenesis II and rapidly increasing breastmilk volume. Engorgement is excessive fullness to the point that the baby can breastfeed only with difficulty. Breasts are warm and feel firm to hard. The mother may have a low-grade fever. (See color plates 59 and 60 in *Clinical lactation: A visual guide*.)

Guidelines for Care

- Frequent breastfeedings—early and often. If infant is sleepy, use rousing techniques to encourage him to feed.
- Express some milk by hand or by pump if the areola/nipple is too hard for infant to grasp. Express after feedings if needed. Use gentle, circular breast massage to assist in leakage.
- Reassure the mother that breast fullness is a positive, healthy sign for breastfeeding and that the breasts will become soft again in time.
- Use a mild analgesic such as ibuprofen or acetaminophen, if needed.
- Take a warm shower. Express milk to relieve fullness while water is running over shoulders and onto breasts.

Finger-Feeding

Infants who are unable to breastfeed—owing to hypotonia, lethargy, or strong extensor positioning—can be finger-fed. Finger-feeding is used to deliver sufficient or extra nutriment to the infant through a feeding tube device while stimulating the maternal milk supply. Finger-feeding is also used to help establish effective and rhythmic suck-swallow patterns by first finger-feeding and then putting baby to breast. The idea is to create a behavior-modification situation that shapes the baby's sucking pattern for feeding at the breast. Commercial supplementers or homemade feeders made from a syringe and 5 fr NG tube can be used.

Instructions for Finger-Feeding

- Wash your hands and make sure your nails are short before you begin.
- Wear a rubber latex-free glove or finger cott according to hospital protocol. (Babies do not always respond well to the feel or taste of rubber in their mouths. If the baby refuses to suck when finger-feeding is attempted, and the person finger-feeding is wearing a glove or a finger cott, assume that the baby is rejecting the glove or cott, not the attempt at finger-feeding).
- Place the baby in the football or cradle position, or prop him high in your lap. This may require the use of a pillow in your lap while your legs are elevated on a footstool, in order to keep the baby comfortably in place. If you are using a dropper or syringe, both hands will be needed.
- When using a dropper, avoid squeezing the milk into the baby's mouth. This can cause gagging, aspiration, and other problems, particularly if the baby is not ready to suck

when the milk is squeezed into his mouth. A more appropriate approach is to put a drop or two into the baby's mouth so that the taste of the milk makes the baby start to suck.

- When using a feeding tube device that can be worn around the neck, the tube can be held or taped to the finger. If tape is used, it should be placed back far enough on the finger (usually above the first joint) and tube so that the tape is not drawn into the baby's mouth. Fluid can loosen the tape.

- Use a medium tube when feeding a normal full-term neonate. However, small or large tubing may be necessary, depending on the baby's sucking response and his overall condition.

- Select a finger that is about the same size as the breadth of the mother's nipple.

- Gently rub the baby's lower lip until his mouth opens. Gradually insert the padded side of your finger toward the roof of the baby's mouth, letting baby pull it in.

- Place the pad side of the provider's finger in the baby's mouth past the alveolar ridge (gum line) but not so deep in his mouth that it triggers the gag reflex. In most instances, the baby will begin suckling as soon as he feels the finger pad on the hard palate.

- If the baby is suckling effectively, the person who is finger-feeding the baby will feel a pulling sensation along the nail bed with each exertion of negative pressure (suckle), as if the nail is being pulled deeper into the baby's mouth, and then feel a reduction of such pressure when the baby swallows. The suck-swallow pattern will be rhythmic.

- Record the amount of human milk (or formula) that the baby takes with each finger-feeding. Neonates should be offered 1–2 ounces with each such feeding. Many times, the baby will take some but not this entire amount. By offering a bit more than you expect the baby will take, you prevent him from sucking air through the tube after he has drained all of the milk from the container.

- Record the baby's response to finger-feeding, including his willingness to do so, his suck pattern, the duration of rhythmic suckling, the presence (if any) of nonrhythmic suckling, and any difficulties the baby exhibited.
- After showing the mother how to finger-feed, help her to learn how to do so, particularly if you anticipate that the baby may need more finger-feedings, or they are likely to occur when you are not available to assist.

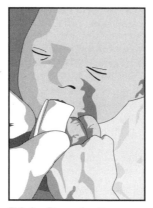

FIG 8   Finger-feeding.

Formula and Non-Human Milk Feedings

All formulas prepared especially for the infant are combinations of fats, protein, carbohydrates, vitamins, and minerals, supplying 20 calories per ounce. They are formulated to be as close as possible to human milk. However, human milk contains many protective factors that cannot be reproduced in infant formula. Cow's milk-based formula contains the same type of nutrients as in cow's milk, but the nutrients have been modified.

Commercial formulas are available in powder, concentrate, and ready-to-feed. If available, mother's own breastmilk can be added to any of these, following mixing or dilution.

Powdered: Least expensive. Use one scoop for every 60 ml of water.

Concentrate: More expensive than powder. Dilute with equal parts of water. Can be stored in the refrigerator for 24 hours. After 24 hours, discard.

Ready-to-feed. Easiest to use and most expensive. The desired amount is poured into a bottle. It can be refrigerated up to 24 hours. After 24 hours, discard.

NUTRITIONAL RECOMMENDATIONS FOR MILK AND FORMULAS

NUTRITIONAL SOURCE	*RECOMMENDATIONS*
Breastmilk added to infant formula	Mother's own milk can be added in order to give the infant his mother's immunity and protective factors. "Inoculating" formula feedings with breastmilk or colostrum is done when there is insufficient volume to give breastmilk alone.
Whole cow's milk	Whole cow's milk is never appropriate for infant in the first six months of life; such feeding may cause enteric bleeding.
Evaporated milk	Evaporated milk does not meet the minimum standards set by the Infant Formula Act. Even when evaporated milk is correctly diluted and mixed with carbohydrate, the infant must be given additional iron and vitamins and the levels of minerals are higher than those in breastmilk.
Skim milk	Defatted milks (2 percent, skim) should not be fed to infants. Infants on skim milk diets gain weight poorly and their skin-fold thickness is inadequate.

Cow's milk-based formula (Similac, Enfamil)	Fat is removed and replaced with soy, oleic, or coconut oil. The protein source is nonfat milk and whey. Lactose is the carbohydrate source. Most cow's milk formula is available with added iron. With mixed bottle and breastfeedings, it is preferable not to use formula with iron as it diminishes the protective effect of lactoferrin in human milk.
Soy-based formula (ProSobee, Nursoy, Soyalac, Isomil, Isomil SF)	Soy-based formula is used for infants who have a temporary lactase deficiency secondary to diarrheas and or galactosemia (very rare). Their fat source is soy oil, oleo, or coconut oil, the protein source is soy protein instead of nonfat milk. Sucrose (table sugar) and corn syrup are used in place of lactose (milk sugar).
Preterm formula (Preemie SMA, Similac Special Care 20 and 24, Enfamil Premature Formula 20 and 24)	Preterm infants need feedings that can support rapid growth without stressing their metabolic and excretory systems. Premature formulas are whey-based because whey contains more cystine. A combination of several carbohydrate and fat sources proved a variety of digestive enzymes for the infant's limited digestive abilities. The vitamin and mineral levels are higher than full-term formula.

Fortifiers, Human Milk

Fortifiers added to human milk provide additional nutrients and accelerate growth in very low birth weight infants, <1500 gm or <1800 gm. The use of fortifiers is associated with hard stools and other symptoms of reduced gastrointestinal tolerance of human milk feeding.

Liquid (Similac Natural Care)	• Provides additional volume and nutrients. Fewer calories, phosphorus, and calcium than powdered fortifier. Has lower osmolarity and renal solute load than powdered fortifier. • Add directly to mother's expressed breastmilk. • Full fortification is 1:1 concentration.
Powdered (Enfamil Human Milk Fortifier or HMF)	• Provides additional nutrients (Ca, phosphorus, ferrous sulfate) and calories but no additional volume. • Developed to mimic pregnancy as Ca and phosphorus levels are plentifully laid down during the last trimester. • HMF added once infant is on full oral feedings. • Warm human milk under running water. Add the powdered fortifier and gently shake. Can be difficult to dissolve.

- A typical order may begin with 2 packets per 100 ml and progress to 3 and then full fortification of 4 packets per 100 ml.
- HMF is made with cow protein, and infant may show signs of intolerance. In such cases, Progestimil is usually substituted. Nutrition services calculate the per-pint ratio of breastmilk: Progestimil.

The following table shows the milk volume needed to meet estimated daily nutrient requirements per kilograms of infant body mass. An infant would need to consume 176 ml of breastmilk per kilogram/day in order to consume the requirement of 120 kcal/kg/day. With fortified milk, the infant could obtain less volume (e.g. 146 or 160 ml) and meet the caloric requirement (manufacturer's product information, Biancuzzo 1999).

Problems with HMF: If mother is only able to produce small amounts of breastmilk or if the baby is requiring small amounts (example 60 ml/24 hr), breastmilk is wasted because the powder is to be added to 25 ml or 50 ml of breastmilk.

MILK VOLUME NEEDED TO MEET ESTIMATED DAILY REQUIREMENTS PER KILOGRAM OF INFANT WEIGHT

Nutrient	Estimated Daily Requirements per Kilogram	Human Milk Only	Human Milk Plus 4 Packets of HMF/100 ml	Human Milk Fortified with Natural Care (1:1 Dilution)
Kilocalories	120 kcal	176 ml	146	160
Protein	≥3 g	286	171	184
Calcium	200 mg	714	169	201
Phosphorus	100 mg	714	169	202
Sodium	2 mEq	256	183	174
Potassium	2 mEq	149	141	99

Galactologues

Occasionally, a medication may be needed to stimulate the mother's milk supply. Galactologues temporarily increase breastmilk volume by blocking dopamine, thus increasing prolactin. They are especially helpful for mothers of premature infants who, in spite of pumping, experience decreasing milk production. Reglan is the most frequently used galactologue in the United States. Domperidone (Motilium), also a dopamine antagonist, is a popular galactologue in Canada.

MEDICATIONS USED TO INCREASE BREASTMILK VOLUME

Domperidone (Motilium)	10 mg orally 3–4 times daily	• Available in Canada only. • Proven useful as a galactologue. • Increases prolactin levels. • Acts primarily in the peripheral dopamine receptor in the GI wall and nausea center in the brain. Minimal crossing of the blood-brain barrier and thus less depression.
Metoclopramide (Reglan)	10 mg orally 3 times daily for 7 to 14 days.	• Small amounts enter into the milk but have not been associated with side effects in the infant. • Maternal depression is a significant side effect. If depression occurs, the drug must be discontinued. • Other maternal side effects include dizziness, nausea, and sweating.
Sulpride (Dolmatil, Sulparex, Sulpitil)	50 mg orally 2–3 times daily	• Major increases in prolactin levels but only moderate increases in breastmilk. Not available in the United States.

Hepatitis B (HBV), Hepatitis C (HCV), Herpes

	GENERAL INFORMATION	BREAST FEED?	RECOMMENDATIONS
Hepatitis B	Can cause systemic illness (fever, fatigue); transmitted by contact with infected blood, body secretions, or blood transfusion. Infants born to HBV-positive mothers are already exposed; most are infected in utero.	Yes	• Can breastfeed after the infant receives hepatitis B vaccine. The infant should receive hepatitis B immunoglobulin (HBIG) before hospital discharge.

(continued)

61

	GENERAL INFORMATION	BREAST FEED?	RECOMMENDATIONS
Hepatitis C	HCV is associated with 80% of non-A, non-B posttransfusion hepatitis. Infants of HCV-infected mothers are already exposed to HCV through exposure to maternal blood during delivery. HCV can be detected in saliva and in breastmilk.	Yes	• Permitted if titers are not high. • Amount in colostrum may be so low as to be unable to infect the newborn infant. • The time amount of HCV present in colostrum may be easily inactivated in the GI tract. • The integrity of the oral and GI mucosa may effectively preclude HCV infection via the oral route (Ho-Hsiung 1995).

| Herpes Simplex 11 | Herpes lesions are painful, blisterlike vesicles and can appear hours to 20 days after exposure. Neonatal infection is usually acquired through infected genital tract. A Cesarean section is usually done when an active lesion is present. Neonates acquiring herpes may become seriously ill. Beyond the first week of life, healthy infants have few adverse effects. | Yes | • Permitted if no lesions on the mother's breast.
 • If mother is mechanically expressing her milk, sterilize all pump parts that are in contact with her skin or her milk after each use.
 • If herpes lesion is not on the breast, the infant may breastfeed provided the mother uses scrupulous hand-washing, gowning, and covering any lesions.
 • Medications and treatment for herpes infections include:
    Acyclovir (Zovirax) orally or topically
    Vidarabine
    Cleanse affected area with Betadine
    Vitamin C and lysine supplements |

HIV/AIDS

General information:

Annually, about 2,000 HIV-infected infants are born in the United States. The rate of HIV infection in women and infants is increasing faster than in any other group. Maternal risk factors include IV drug use and sexual contact with a partner who is an IV drug user or is bisexual and has AIDS.

Additionally, an infant born to an infected mother has an 8–18% chance of developing AIDS if breastfeeding. Infants infected with HIV appear to be slower to develop symptoms of AIDS if they are breastfed.

Guidelines for care

- There is risk of transmitting HIV to the infant through breastmilk if an at-risk mother seroconverts to HIV+ status very late in her pregnancy or early postpartum while she is lactating.
- About one-third of infants born to healthy HIV+ mothers worldwide will become infected regardless of how they are fed. Two-thirds of infants born to HIV+ mothers will not seroconvert to HIV+ status.
- Gloves are usually not used unless the worker frequently handles breastmilk, as in a milk bank. Breastmilk is not included in mandatory universal precautions recommendations.
- A healthy HIV+ mother who wishes to provide her baby with breastmilk can do so if that milk is pasteurized; pasteurization kills the human immunodeficiency virus.

Hindmilk, Feedings

Foremilk is that milk that is expressed in the first stage of pumping; hindmilk is the milk obtained during the later half of pumping. The purpose of hindmilk feedings is to concentrate the natural fat in mother's milk so those premature infants can receive extra calories without extra milk volume. By fractionating the hindmilk portion of a milk expression, mothers can provide a high-lipid, high-calorie milk that promotes accelerated infant growth. Low birth weight infants have been shown to gain significantly more weight when given concentrated hindmilk feedings (Valentine et al. 1994).

Hindmilk and foremilk portions of a given pumping session are not clearly delineated; rather, hindmilk has a higher concentration of milk fat than does foremilk, which has a higher protein portion. Separating foremilk from hindmilk thus increases the concentration of fats but does not preclude the inclusion of milk fat in the earlier expressed foremilk portion.

Guidelines for Collecting Hindmilk

1. Have two containers available, each marked with a color or labeled for foremilk and hindmilk. Label containers with the infant's and mother's name, time, and date of expression and the baby's identification number. Option: Red (foremilk), indication not to use, freeze until the infant is discharged; yellow (hindmilk), refrigerate or freeze milk until it is transported to the hospital for infant feeding.
2. The milk from each pumping must be kept in its own container and not mixed with milk from other pumpings. Store the milk in feeding-sized portions.

65

3. Place collection devices on the breast, taking care not to touch the flange area.
4. Use the breast pump. Encourage the mother to touch, hold, or think about the infant during pumping to maximize milk volume and letdown. If she has a free hand, she should be encouraged to touch or hold the baby while she is pumping the breast.
5. Two minutes after the milk starts to flow steadily, stop pumping. Place the first milk obtained into the container labeled "Foremilk."
6. Resume pumping again and continue for up to two minutes after milk is no longer being expressed from the breasts. The last few drops of milk obtained contain the most fat. Place this portion of the milk in the container labeled "Hindmilk."
7. The milk may be refrigerated or frozen at home or brought to the nursery to be used or stored as needed for the individual mother and infant.
8. Sterilize all milk collection equipment once daily, either by boiling for 20 minutes or in the dishwasher with a sani-cycle. Wash all pumping equipment thoroughly with soap and hot water after each milk expression. Allow equipment to air dry between use.

Immunizations, Infant and Mother

General information:
The Centers for Disease Control (1994) advises that "neither killed nor live vaccines affect the safety of breastfeeding for mothers or infants."

Infant immunization:
• It is recommended that the breastfeeding infant immunization schedule be the same as the formula-feeding baby.
• Studies have found that some immunizations tend to produce a more active immune response if the baby is receiving human milk.

Maternal immunization: Immunization of the mother poses no harm to the healthy, full-term breastfeeding infant. Breastfeeding women can receive an influenza vaccine and RhoGAM without harm to infant.

TYPE OF INFANT IMMUNIZATION	OK TO GIVE	COMMENTS
DPT	Yes	Not altered by breastfeeding.
H. influenzae type b	Yes	Breastfed infants have higher antibody titers than nonbreast-feeding infants.
Hepatitis B	Yes	Not altered by breastfeeding.
MMR (measles, mumps, rubella)	Yes	Virus found in the breastmilk when given to the rubella seronegative woman after birth, poses no risk to infant.
OPV	Yes	It is not necessary to withhold breastfeeding before or after administration of OPV.
Varicella (chickenpox)	Yes	Not altered by breastfeeding.

Inadequate Milk Supply, Actual

General information:

Very few women have a physically based problem (hormone imbalance, previous breast surgery, and breast hypoplasia) that can lead to an insufficient milk supply. In this case, the infant is not gaining weight adequately. Regardless of the appropriate feeding frequency and optimal breastfeeding management, supplementing the infant is necessary.

Assessment:

- Determine if the mother has had breast surgery, what kind, when, and the reasons for it.
- Assess for marked differences in breast size and shape, and for a wide space between the breasts in the absence of injury or surgery to the breast.
- Observe the infant's pattern of breastfeeding. The skills the baby brings to the breastfeeding encounter may be contributing to inadequate milk volume secondary to inadequate or suboptimal breast stimulation.

Guidelines for Care

- Supplement infant feedings with donated or banked human milk or artificial baby milk using a tube/syringe feeding apparatus or cup feeding.
- Determine whether the problem is maternal or infant-related:

  If a maternal cause, determine if that cause can be resolved. If it cannot, provide the mother with this information.

  If an infant cause, determine if that cause can be resolved. In most cases, this can be done with time and patience and

69

maternal willingness to assist the baby to breastfeed more effectively.

Involve the mother in the decision-making process and related resolution of the problem.

Discuss with the mother the appropriateness of continuing the breastfeeding relationship in the face of the need to supplement her milk production.

Inadequate Milk Supply, Perceived

General information:

The most frequently mentioned reason why mothers wean their babies is their belief that they do not have sufficient milk to sustain adequate growth of their infant. This perception may reflect other peoples' views, maternal fears, and/or maternal misunderstanding of how breastfeeding works–for example, when breast fullness subsides and the infant goes through an appetite spurt, thus increasing the frequency of feedings. The mother may conclude that the baby's behavior–wanting to feed more often–is an indication that she is not making enough milk.

Guidelines for Care

- Assess the number of wet diapers. By the end of the first week, the infant should have at least six to eight wet cloth diapers or four to six wet disposable diapers. Assessment in the first week should use the "rule of thumb" of at least one wet diaper for each day of life.
- Assess the number of stools. By the end of the first week, 5–10/day and mostly yellow milk stools should be seen.
- Assess the frequency and effectiveness of feeds to verify that milk transfer is occurring. Infrequent feeds may be reflected in:
  infrequent wet diapers
  infrequent stools
  little or no early weight gain.
- Increasing feeds to 8 or more in 24 hours often resolves the problem within 48 hours.
- Weigh the infant using an electronic scale to determine adequate weight gain. Infants should gain no fewer than 4 to 7 ounces (113 to 219 gm) per week or at least a pound (500 gm) a month after regaining birth

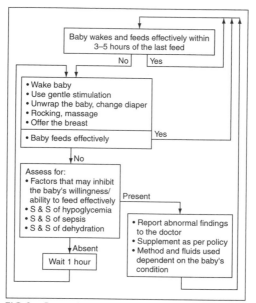

FIG 9   Breastfeeding flowchart.
*Source: Reprinted with permission from Plenum Publishing
Corp. and J. Glover: Supplementation of breastfeeding
newborns: a flowchart for decision-making.* J Hum Lact
11:127–131, 1995.

weight. The infant should have regained
birth weight by the end of two weeks.

- If the infant is receiving sufficient breastmilk
  for growth, reassure the mother that her
  body is adequately nourishing her baby and
  counsel her that:

Breastfed babies feed often because
    breastmilk is easily and quickly digestible.

Appetite spurts cause an infant to *temporarily*
    increase feeding frequency.

Advise the mother to:

- Let the baby finish the first breast before offering the second breast.
- Offer both breasts during each feeding to ensure that the infant has ample opportunity to feed. If the baby prefers one breast only, do not restrict the time on that breast. If the contralateral breast is uncomfortably full, encourage the mother to express milk from the unnursed breast.
- Limiting the duration of feeds can interfere with adequate milk transfer, particularly of hindmilk, which represents the later portion of each feed. The baby is more likely to be satiated when allowed to obtain adequate hindmilk.

Induced Lactation

General information:

A woman who wishes to breastfeed her adopted baby can do so. The key to developing a milk supply is her own motivation to put her baby to breast and the baby's willingness to suckle.

Assessment:

- Take a careful maternal history. Assess the mother's rationale for wishing to induce lactation and how she intends to determine if she is "successful."
- Review the effect of the infant's age and ability and willingness to suckle on the induced lactation process.

Guidelines for Care

- Inform the mother about how she can feed her baby at the breast while simultaneously stimulating her breasts to make milk and protecting the baby's nutritional integrity.
- Inform the mother of the importance of having a breastfeeding relationship irrespective of the volume of milk she will produce.
- Encourage the mother to learn as much about breastfeeding as she can (this is especially important if she has never had a baby) so that she can appropriately assess infant cues to be nurtured and to be fed.
- Be prepared to assure the mother that drugs are not necessary to induce lactation; the most effective means of developing a milk supply is a vigorously sucking infant who loves to breastfeed frequently.
- Consider getting the mother in touch with other mothers who have successfully induced lactation and enjoyed the breastfeeding relationship.

- Remind the mother that her success is unrelated to milk volume or how little supplement her baby may need; rather, her goal should be developing a mutually enjoyable mother-baby relationship.

Infant, Expected Milk Intake

- Assess whether the infant is gaining weight in keeping with expectations for the child's age.
- If the infant is gaining adequately, assure the mother that this is occurring.
- If the infant is not gaining as expected, review those elements related to Inadequate Milk Supply, Actual, on p. 69.

AVERAGE INFANT BREASTMILK INTAKE PER FEEDING

AGE	AMOUNT	
	OZ.	ML
Birth to 24 hrs	1/4	7–14
24 hrs.–2 wks.	1–1.5	30–45
2 wks.–1 mo.	1–3	30–90
1–2 mo.	2–3	60–90
2–4 mo.	3–4	90–120
4–6 mo.	4–5	120–150

ESTIMATES OF INFANT
INTAKE/DAY BY WEIGHT (KG)

WEIGHT		*INTAKE*	
LBS.	*KG.*	*OZ.*	*ML*
5	2.26	13	371
6	2.72	16	457
7	3.17	19	542
8	3.62	21	600
9	4.08	24	685
10	4.53	27	771
11	4.99	29	828
12	5.44	32	914

CAUTION: The above estimate is more easily assessed when a baby is fed by bottle. Assessment at breast can be made with careful before-after weights when using an electronic scale that is carefully calibrated and has a very low rate of error. Estimating by means of observing feeding behavior alone is generally unlikely to provide an accurate estimate of breastmilk intake.

Infant, Insufficient Weight Gain

General information:

Neonates are expected to lose 5–10% of their birth weight after birth. Breastfeeding infants are expected to regain their birth weight by the end of the second week, to double their birth weight at 5–6 months, and to triple their birth weight by one year. Heredity and individual growth patterns affect weight gain.

Breastfed and artificially fed infants are roughly similar in weight and height changes until 3–4 months of age, after which the formula-fed infant begins to add more weight. By age 2 years, weight gain is again similar.

Signs of insufficient weight gain:
- After day 3, the baby is having < 4 wet diapers/day (cloth) and < 3 wet disposable diapers.
- After day 4, the infant is having fewer than 3–4 stools per day.
- Infant has not regained birth weight by the end of the second week.
- After 4 weeks, the infant is gaining less than 4 oz. per week.

Assess the following factors:
- Limited duration of feedings; who is signaling the end of the feeding?
- Excessively long feedings characterized by a baby who appears to "sleep" or "graze" at the breast.
- Limited number of feedings: sleepy, "good" baby, inexperienced mother. In most cases, the baby should have unlimited access to the breast from birth and a minimum of 8–12 vigorous feedings/day after the first week.
- Ineffective positioning of the infant at breast. The infant should be directly facing

mother (chest to chest), with as much of the areola in the infant's mouth as possible.

- Ineffective or disorganized suckling, excessive drawing in of the infant's cheeks, no audible swallowing sounds, infant's eyes closed throughout the feeding, and fussiness after appearing to have fed well.
- Rule out the following conditions in the infant:
Urinary tract infections
Tongue-tie (ankyloglossia)
Inherited metabolic disease
Cardiac disease
Insufficient glandular tissue
Poor letdown
Hypothyroidism
- Rule out the following conditions in the mother:
Insufficient glandular tissue with or without breast hypoplasia
Inadequate or ineffective milk ejection
Hypothyroidism

Guidelines for Care

- Determine if health problems in mother or infant are playing a contributing role in the problem. Correct those problems, if possible.
- Seek a second opinion if the baby has ankyloglossia and where indicated, recommend that the frenulum be clipped. Dentists and oral surgeons will do this when pediatricians hesitate.
- If the infant problem or maternal problem requires drug therapy, assist in recommending medication(s) that are not contraindicated during breastfeeding.
- If health problems in mother or infant or both have been ruled out, refer to Inadequate Milk Supply, Actual, on p. 69 to assess and resolve the problem.

Jaundice

General information:

Most neonatal jaundice is a normal physiologic, protective adjustment to extrauterine life. Higher levels are found in Asian and Native Americans in North America. Jaundice occurs later in preterm infants. There are three types of neonatal jaundice:

Early-Onset (Physiologic) Jaundice in the Term Infant

Onset 2–3 days after birth, usually disappears within 7–10 days, although bilirubin levels may remain elevated for several weeks. Usually peaks 3–5 days after birth < 15 mg/dl. Babies with non-Rh-caused jaundice will tolerate bilirubin levels of 23–29 mg/dl without a risk of kernicterus. The condition is related to insufficient intake of human milk and/or delayed and infrequent breastfeeding.

Guidelines for Care

- Encourage continued frequent feedings at the breast. Colostrum/breastmilk has a laxative effect, stimulating the passage of meconium and thus lowering peak bilirubin levels.
- If temporary supplements are needed, calorie-dense, milk-based fluids–not water or glucose water–should be used.
- Phototherapy is not indicated unless the serum bilirubin is above 20 mg/dl and is continuing to rise after day 3.

Late-Onset (Breastmilk) Jaundice

Occurs after the first week of life and persists > 1 month. This is thought to be a rare occurrence. The peak varies: Bilirubin levels may exceed 20 mg/dl. Inhibitors in breastmilk or immaturity of the infant's liver or both may cause condition.

Guidelines for Care

- There is no need to interrupt breastfeeding if the bilirubin level is below 25 in the first 14 days and baby is feeding well and voiding and stooling appropriately for age.

If bilirubin level is above 25 mg/dl after 14 days:
- Alternate breast and formula feeds for 24 hours or temporarily interrupt breastfeeding for 24 hours, and ask the mother to express her milk. Supplements should be milk other than the mother's.
- Return to breastfeeding; expect a slight rebound in continued bilirubin levels, followed by a gradual decline in those levels, sometimes as late as 4 months of life.

Pathologic Jaundice

Onset of rapidly rising bilirubin levels within the first day postpartum.

Guidelines for Care

- Assess for hemolytic diseases of the newborn (ABO or Rh incompatibilities), infections, diabetes, or organic disease.
- Surgery, phototherapy, or exchange transfusion may be required.
- Encourage the mother to continue breastfeeding frequently or pumping if the baby is taken off the breast throughout the period of additional therapy.

Mastitis

General information:

The most frequently identified pathogen is *staphylococcus aureus*. If infectious mastitis, the milk may taste salty from higher levels of sodium and chloride and simultaneously reduced milk flow. The mother should continue breastfeeding. Antibiotics (penicillin-resistant) are usually given. Rarely beta hemolytic streptococcus, E. coli, and H. influenzae may be involved. (See color plate 66 in *Clinical lactation: A visual guide*.)

Symptoms of noninfectious mastitis:
- Mother notes a "hot spot" or area of acute tenderness.
- Mother may feel a small, hard area in the area of tenderness.
- Mother does not have a fever and feels well.

Symptoms of infectious mastitis:
- Mother complains of fatigue and flulike muscular aches.
- Mother may complain of a headache.
- Mother has a fever above 101°F (34°C).
- The breast may have a circumscribed or more extensive area of soreness.
- The breast may have a red streak tender and/or hard to the touch.
- The skin of the breast may appear to be red or shiny (a late sign).
- The entire breast may feel hard and tight and she may describe this as "engorgement."

Factors often contributing to mastitis:
- Nipple cracks or fissures
- History of mastitis
- Poor feeding by baby
- Infrequent offering of the breast
- Fatigue and stress

Guidelines for Care:

- Prescribe antistaphylococcal antibiotics (dicloxacillin 125 mg 4x/day for 7 days) unless fever and symptoms are already subsiding.
- Continue breastfeeding.
- Apply moist heat to sore area.
- Bedrest (with infant) as much as possible.
- Non-narcotic analgesic, antipyretic (ibuprofen, acetaminophen) to reduce fever and pain.
- Monitor body temperature for fever. If the mother has a high fever, <102°F, culture milk for possibility of streptococcal infection.
- Early intervention is usually effective in preventing breast abscess.
- Culture for causative organism if the mother has repeated episodes of mastitis.
- If repeated episodes, consider a blockage of the duct indicative of a galactocele, cyst, or tumor.

SELECTED ANTIBIOTICS FOR MASTITIS

Generic Name	*Trade Name*	*Adult Dosage Ranges*
Penicillinase-Resistant Penicillins		
Cloxacillin	Cloxapen, Tegopen	250–500 mg PO q6h
Dicloxacillin	Dynapen	125–250 mg PO or IM q6h
Oxacillin	Prostaphlin	500 mg–1 gram PO or IM q4-6h
Cephalosporins		
Cephalexin	Keflex	250–500 mg PO q6h
Cepharadine	Anspor, Velosef	250–500 mg PO q6h
Cefaclor	Ceclor	250–500 mg PO q8h

Other

Erythromycin	E-mycin	250–500 mg PO q6h
		If allergic to penicillin or as preventative for recurring infections
Nasal mupirocin	Bactroban (ointment)	Nasal application may help reduce carrier state

Medications, Maternal

General information:

Although the placenta permits a ready crossover of drugs to the fetus in utero, the breast serves as a formidable barrier against such transmission that protects the infant. Most drugs pass through to the mother's milk but they do so in minute amounts, usually less than 1% of the maternal dose. Most are not harmful to the infant; many cannot be found when infant serum is checked.

Guidelines for Care

The goal is to *assist the mother to continue breast-feeding.*

- Use a medication only if it is necessary. In some cases the mother may not need the medication. Consider alternative nondrug therapies.
- Delay suggesting use of a medication (if there is a choice) until the infant is maturer and better able to detoxify and metabolize drugs that might be transported through the milk. This is especially important if the baby is preterm.
- Suggest the lowest dose possible for the shortest time possible.
- Recommend using a drug that transfers the least amount into breastmilk, using its reported milk/plasma ratio as a guide. Avoid drugs with an M/P greater than or equal to 1.
- Avoid medications with a long half-life or those with sustained release preparations.
- Recommend scheduling the medication dose so that the lowest amount gets into the milk—usually immediately after a feeding or before the infant has a long sleep period.

- Ask the mother to observe for any untoward reaction, such as infant fussiness, rash, colic, or any marked change in feeding or sleeping habits. If any of these occur, the physician should be notified and informed about all of the medications being used by the mother.
- Offer instructions for expressing her milk if the mother must take a drug that is contraindicated for a short time during breastfeeding. Reassure her that breastfeeding can continue after the medication in question is no longer needed.

MEDICATIONS USED BY BREASTFEEDING WOMEN

Aspirin and NSAIDs

Aspirin
Acetaminophen (Tylenol)
Ibuprofen (Motrin, Advil)

Narcotics/Analgesics

Codeine
Oxycodon (Percadon)
Propoxyphene (Darvocet)
Hydrocodone (Lortab, Vicodin)

Antibiotics

Amoxicillin
Ampicillin
Azithromycin (Zithromax)
Dicloxicillin

Antibiotics (continued)

Metronidazole (Flagyl)*
Penicillin

Antihistamines/Decongestants

Claratin
Dimetapp*
Robitussin
Pseudoephedrine (Sudafed, Actifed)

Antifungals

Clotrimazole (Gyne-Lotrimin)
Fluconazole (Diflucan)
Monistat
Nystatin

Anti-ulcer

Prilosec
Famotidine (Pepcid)

Laxatives/Stool softeners

Bisacodyl (Dulcolax)
Docusate (Colace)
Metamucil
Mylicon

Antidepressants

Amitriptyline (Elavil)*
Desipramine (Norpramine)
Sertraline (Zoloft)
Fluoxetine (Prozac)*

Antidepressants (continued)

Paroxetine (Paxil)
St. John's Wort
Diazepam (Valium)

Antidiarrheal

Loperamide (Maalox, Immodium)

Antihypertensives

Atenolol (Tenormin)*

Contraceptives

Depo-Provera
Norplant

(continued)

MEDICATIONS USED BY BREASTFEEDING WOMEN

Contraceptives (continued)

Oral contraceptives, combined*

Oral contraceptives, progestin only (Micronor)

Bronchial Dilators

Albuterol inhaler (Proventil, Ventolin)

Synthroid

Vitamins

Vaccines

* Indicates caution. Another drug should be considered.

GUIDE FOR MEDICATIONS AND BREASTFEEDING

A = Relatively safe; B = Use with caution; C = Unknown; D = Contraindicated

MEDICATION	A	B	C	D	COMMENTS
Acetaminophen (Tylenol)	√				• Non-narcotic analgesic. Used postpartum.
Acyclovir (Zovirax)	√				• Used for herpes. Low concentrations in milk.
Albuterol (Proventil)	√				• Inhaled: Less than 10% is absorbed. Not likely to produce clinically relevant levels in breastfed infants. Oral: Breastmilk levels could be sufficient to produce tremors or agitation in infants.
Alprazolam (Xanax)			√		• Use alternate drug. Risk of accumulation.
Amantadine (Symmetrel)	√				• Small insignificant levels in breastmilk. Given directly to children after age 1.
Aminophylline	√				• Observe infant for irritability and insomnia.
Ampicillin	√				• Passes into milk in low concentrations.

(continued)

MEDICATION	A	B	C	D	COMMENTS
Amitriptyline (Elavil)	√				• No drug detected in infant's urine.
Amoxicillin	√				• Used for otitis media in children. Less than 0.7% of maternal dose is transferred to breastmilk.
Aspirin	√				• Usual analgesic dose (300–600 mg) is probably safe. Drug of choice for long-term arthritis treatment.
Atenolol (Tenormin)		√			• One report of infant cyanosis and bradycardia with maternal therapy.
Azithromycin	√				• Small insignificant levels in breastmilk.
Bromocriptine (Parlodel)				√	• Not to be used for suppressing breastmilk supply.
Brompheniramine (Dimetane, Dimetapp)		√			• Reported cases of irritability, excessive crying, and reduction in milk supply.
Butorphanol (Stadol)	√				• Safe in single doses. Sedation possible in neonates.
Caffeine	√				• Infant irritability and wakefulness if maternal dose is high.

Captopril (Capoten)	√	• Antihypertensive. Minute amounts in milk.
Carbamazepine (Tegretol)	√	• Anticonvulsant. No apparent accumulation.
Cephalosporins (Cefaclor, Cefamandole, Cefazolin, Cefixime, Cefotaxime, Cefoxitin, Cephalexin)	√	• Passes into breast milk in low concentrations. Generally considered safe.
Choramphenicol (Chloromycetin)		√ • Small risk of bone marrow suppression. Adverse effects reported.
Chloroquine (Aralen)	√	• Antimalarial. Minute amounts in milk.
Chlorpromazine (Thorazine)	√	• Tranquilizer. Drug has long half-life. Observe infant for sedation.
Cimetidine (Tagamet)		√ • H-2 antagonist, decreases acid production.

(continued)

93

MEDICATION	A	B	C	D	COMMENTS
Ciprofloxacin (Cipro)			√		• Fluoroquinolone antibiotic. Amount present in breast-milk is low. Requires a risk/benefit assessment. Associated with arthropathy in adolescent children.
Clindamycin (Cleocin)	√				• Vaginal cream, oral and injectionable form.
Clotrimazole (Gyne-Lotrimin)	√				• Used for candidiasis. Unlikely that levels absorbed by infant would be high enough for adverse effects.
Codeine	√				• Commonly used for postpartum pain. Safe for healthy term infants in short-term use. Infant receives approx. 0.1% of maternal dose.
Contraceptives, oral progestin only	√				• Wait until lactation is established, 4–6 weeks.
Contraceptives, oral (with estrogen)				√	• Will reduce milk supply.
Crotamiton 10%	√				• Used for scabies. Safe and effective for lactating women.

Corticosteroids (ACTH, Prednisone)	√	• Use for short periods with low dose only.
Desipramine (Norpramin)	√	• No drug detected in infant's urine.
Diazepam (Valium)		√ • Use alternate drug. Risk of accumulation.
Dicloxacillin	√	• Used to treat mastitis. Minute amounts in breastmilk.
Digoxin (Lanoxin)	√	• Antiarrhythmic drug. Exposure to infant insignificant.
Ergotamine		√ • Used for migraines. Suppresses milk supply. May cause vomiting, diarrhea, convulsions.
Erythromycin (E-mycin)	√	• Commonly used in children over 1 month of age.
Ethosuximide (Zarontin)		√ • Anticonvulsant. Passes freely into breastmilk. Consider using alternate drug.
Fentanyl (Sublimaze)	√	• Appears in small amounts in breastmilk. Undetectable after 10 hrs.
Fluconazole (Diflucan)	√	• Used to treat candidiasis. Safe for pediatric use.
Fluoxetine (Prozac)		√ • May cause colicky symptoms.

(continued)

MEDICATION	A	B	C	D	COMMENTS
Furosemide (Lasix)	√				• Antibiotic aminoglycoside. Can be given to infants.
Gentamicin (Garamycin)	√				• Minimal transfer.
Heparin	√				• Not excreted into breastmilk.
Ibuprofen (Motrin)	√				• Commonly used for postpartum pain. Minimal transfer.
Imipramine (Trofanil)	√				• Antidepressant. Minimal transfer to breastmilk.
Influenza vaccine	√				• Maternal vaccination does not present risk to nursing infant.
Insulin	√				• Not excreted into breastmilk due to high molecular weight.
Iodide			√		• Readily absorbed and concentrated in breastmilk; could cause thyroid suppression; 15% of dose passed into milk in three days.
Iron	√				• Supplementation does not appreciably change iron levels in milk.

Drug		Comments
Isoniazid (INH)	√	Antitubercular. No infant adverse effects reported to date. May be prudent to monitor infants for signs of toxicity.
Ketoconazole (Nizoral)	√	Used to treat severe candidiasis. Fluconazole preferred for lactating women.
Levonogestrel (NORPLANT)	√	Contraceptive. Effect on milk supply inconclusive. Level of progestin in infant approx. 10% of maternal circulation.
Lindane (Kwell)	√	Clinically insignificant (30ng/mL) amounts in breast-milk. Need more information.
Lithium (Eskalith)	√	Monitor infant's serum levels. Choose alternative drug if possible.
Magnesium sulfate	√	Delays lactogenesis following birth. Amount in breastmilk not clinically relevant.

MEDICATION	A	B	C	D	COMMENTS
Medroxyprogesterone (Depo-Provera)	√				• Insignificant amounts transfer into breastmilk. Anecdotal reports of decline in milk supply following injection.
Meperidine (Demerol)				√	• May cause neurobehavioral depression and ineffective suckling.
Mesoridazine (Serentil)	√				• Phenothiazine used as antipsychotic.
Metaproterenol (Alupent)			√		• Used for bronchial asthma.
Metformin (Glucophage)			√		• Oral hypoglycemic agent for diabetics. Due to low protein binding and low molecular weight, other oral hypoglycemics are preferred.
Methadone (Dolophine)	√				• Used to treat heroin addiction. Small amounts transfer into breastmilk. AAP approves use if dose <20 mg/24 hrs.
Methimazole (Tapazol)	√				• For hyperthyroidism. M:P ratio higher than propyl-thiouracil.

Methyldopa (Aldomet)	√	• Antihypertensive. Levels transferred to breastfeeding infant too low for clinical significance.
Metoclopramide (Reglan)	√	• Used to increase breastmilk; dose: 10 mg t.i.d.
Metoprolol (Lopressor)		√ • Due to blocking action, monitor infant if using long term.
Morphine	√	• Safe for short-term use for pain control. Infants are more alert and better oriented than if the mother receives meperidine.
Nadolol (Corgard)		√ • Avoid if young infant and/or high doses needed.
Nalbuphine (Nubain)	√	• Narcotic analgesia. Safe in single doses.
Naproxen (Naprosen)	√	• Passes into breastmilk in small quantities (0.26% of maternal dose).
Nifedipine	√	• Low doses used to treat nipple vasospasm. <5% of maternal dose transfers to infant.

(continued)

MEDICATION	A	B	C	D	COMMENTS
Nitrofurantoin	√				• Used for treating urinary tract infections. Trace amounts in breastmilk.
Nortriptyline (Pamelor)	√				• Used to treat postpartum depression. Milk levels are low to undetectable.
Nystatin (Mycostatin)	√				• Safe. Used for candidiasis.
Ofloxacin (Floxin)			√		• Fluoroquinolone antibiotic similar to ciprofloxacin. Levels in breastmilk are consistently lower (37%) than ciprofloxacin.
Oxycodone (Percodan)	√				• Commonly used for postpartum pain. Safe for short-term use.
Paroxetine (Paxil)			√		• Popular antidepressant. <1% of daily dose transferred to breastfeeding infant.
Penicillin (Pen G, Pen V)	√				• Excreted into breastmilk in low concentrations. Modi-fication bowel flora and allergenic response possible.

Drug		Comments
Phenazopyridine (Pyridium)	•	Used for urinary tract disease. May cause discoloring of breastmilk.
Phenytoin (Dilantin)	✓	Used for control of seizure disorders. Levels in breastmilk <5% of therapeutic dose for infants.
Polophyllin	✓	Used for treatment of genital warts. Do not use during lactation.
Propoxyphene (Darvon)	✓	Narcotic analgesic. Used for postpartum pain. Minimal amounts in breastmilk.
Propranolol (Inderal)	✓	Popular beta blocker for treating hypertension. Small amounts in breastmilk are clinically insignificant. Preferred beta blocker for lactation.
Propylthiouracil	✓	For treating hyperthyroidism. Infant receives only 0.025% of maternal dose. Preferred medication for lactation.
Pyrethrins	✓	Used to treat pediculosis. Topical absorption poor. Low potential for toxicity. Preferred to Lindane.

(continued)

Medication	A	B	C	D	Comments
Quinidine	√				• Antiarrhythmic drug.
Ranitidine (Zantac)	√				• Infant receives very small amounts in breastmilk.
Rifampin (Rimactane)	√				• Antitubercular. No adverse effects have been reported.
Sertraline (Zoloft)	√				• Popular antidepressant. Not detected in infant serum. No untoward effects noted in studies.
Sotalol (Betapace)			√		• Passes into milk in relatively high amounts, although no adverse effects have been reported. Monitor infant for side effects.
Stool softeners and bulk-forming laxatives	√				• Local effect.
Streptomycin			√		• Given to infants directly. Not to be given for longer than two weeks.
Sulfonamides			√		• Avoid during first month of life. Displaces bilirubin.

Sulpride	√	• Increases prolactin levels and breastmilk production. Small doses effective for insufficient milk supply. Not available in the USA.
Tamoxifen		√ • Anticancer drug. Long half-life. Inhibits lactation. Risks outweigh benefits.
Terbutaline (Brethaire)	√	• Infant's dose 0.2% of maternal dose. Symptoms of beta-adrenergic stimulation not noted in any of study infants.
Terconazole (Terazol)	√	• Used for candidiasis. Vaginal cream and suppositories.
Terfenadine (Seldane)	√	• Antihistamine. Estimated amounts consumed by neonate after mother given recommended dose are not likely to result in plasma level producing untoward effects.
Tetracycline	√	• Minimal amounts transferred into breastmilk. Compatible with breastfeeding for short terms.

(continued)

MEDICATION	A	B	C	D	COMMENTS
Theophylline (Aminophylline)	√				• Less than 0.1% is absorbed by infant. May occasionally cause irritability in newborns.
Thioridazine (Mellaril)	√				• Phenothiazine used as antipsychotic.
Thyroid and thyroxine (Synthroid)			√		• May improve milk volume if mother is hypothyroid.
Verapamil (Isoptin)	√				• No drug detected in plasma of infants.

Derived from: American Academy of Pediatrics Committee on Drugs, "Transfer of Drugs and Other Chemicals into Human Milk," *Pediatrics* 93 (1994); G. C. Briggs, et al., *Drugs in Pregnancy and Lactation*, 5th ed. (Baltimore: Williams & Wilkins, 1998); T. Hale, *Clinical Therapy in Breastfeeding Patients*. (Amarillo, TX: Pharmasoft Medical Publishing, 1999); T. Hale, *Medications and Mothers' Milk*, 8th ed. (Amarillo, TX: Pharmasoft Medical Publishing, 1999); R. Lawrence, *Breastfeeding: A Guide for the Medical Profession*, 5th ed. (St. Louis: Mosby 1999).

Milk Banks

The following are donor human milk banks in North America which collect, screen, process, store, and distribute donated human milk. A physician prescription is required.

Banco De Leche, Dr. Rafael Lucio
Xalapa, Veracruz, Mexico
52-55-14-45-10 EXT. 204
Fax: 52-55-14-45-51

Lactation Support Services
British Columbia Childrens' Hospital
Vancouver, BC CANADA
604-875-2345

Mothers' Milk Bank
Columbia/ Presbyterian/ St Luke's Medical Center
1719 E. 19th Ave
Denver, CO
303-998-4550

Mothers' Milk Bank at Austin
900 E. 30th St., Suite 101
Austin, TX 78705
512-494-0800

Regional Milk Bank
Medical Center of Central Massachusetts
Worcester, MA
508-793-6005

Lactation Center and Mothers' Milk Bank at
   WakeMed
Wake Medical Center
Raleigh, NC
919-350-8599

Wilmington Mothers' Milk Bank
Christiana Care Health System
Wilmington, DE
310-733-2340

Nipple, Blister ("Bleb")

General information:

Whitish, tender area where a small amount of milk becomes lodged under the epidermis and triggers an inflammatory response. This condition may be associated with a plugged duct.

Guidelines for Care

- Attempt to manually compress with a clean diaper or sterile gauze before breastfeeding. Doing so in a shower often works well. This may open the blister.
- Alternate the infant's position at breast.
- Open and aspirate the blister with sterile needle using sterile procedure (physician or advanced practice provider). Encourage immediate expression to obtain full free flow of milk from the affected duct. Apply a topical antibiotic.
- Use breast shell or sore nipple inserts which protects the nipple/areola tissue during the initial tender period after opening the affected area. Air holes in the shell will provide air circulation to enhance healing.
- Suggest temporary expression of milk if the mother is in extreme pain. Return to full breastfeeding as soon as this is possible.

Nipple, Leaking

General information:
Leaking from the breasts is normal and helps to relieve fullness in the early postpartum period. Stimuli that may trigger leaking include a crying infant, sexual intercourse, and full breasts. Occasionally a woman will have an unexplained episode of breast fullness and leaking long after she has weaned.

Guidelines for Care

- Feed the baby frequently (or express milk) to keep the breasts from becoming uncomfortably full.
- Use nursing pads or other absorbent material (100% cotton is preferred) to absorb milk leakage. Change pads after each feeding.
- Temporarily reduce leakage by pressing the palm of the hand flat on the nipple.
- Wear print or patterned colors to hide leaks on clothing.

Nipple, Shields

Nipple shields are thin silicone devices shaped like a nipple and are worn over the mother's nipple during feedings. Shields can be helpful but their continued use harbors a risk that the infant will imprint on the shield and refuse the breast. Decrease in milk intake can also be a risk factor in some cases.

Indications for using nipples shields are:

- inverted nipples
- difficulties in latch-on and suckling
- engorgement
- extremely forceful letdowns
- very sore nipples
- making the "switch" to breastfeeding after bottle-feeding

Guidelines for Use

- Wash hands well and clean the shield with hot, soapy water.
- Dampen the shield with a small amount of breastmilk or water.
- Place the shield over the breast with the nipple in the center of the shield.
- Lightly touch the shield to the baby's lips to stimulate latch-on with a wide gap.
- Encourage suckling.
- Evaluate milk transfer by listening for audible swallowing and asking the mother if she feels a letdown.
- Weigh the infant every week on an electronic scale to assess for adequate weight gain.

Weaning from the Shield

- Feed the infant before he gets hungry so he is less likely to become impatient with weaning from the shield.

- Carry out weaning attempts during baby's "happiest" time of the day.
- Start the feeding with the shield for 2–3 minutes, then quickly remove it and latch the baby on again.

In the event that the baby refuses to suckle the breast without the shield, assess for adequacy of weight gain and frequency of feedings. If weight gain is age-appropriate and the mother is feeding frequently, reassure her that she can continue to breastfeed with the shield.

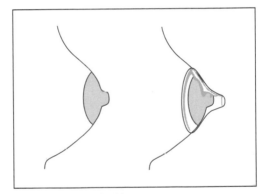

FIG 10   Nipple shield.

Nipples, Sore

Transient: The majority of new mothers develop a transient soreness of their nipples that does not last beyond the first 7–10 days postpartum. Peak soreness usually occurs 3–7 days postpartum and resolves after the first week. (See color plates 61, 62, 63, and 64 in Clinical lactation: A visual guide.) Reassure the mother that the nipple soreness is temporary. Less than 10% of mothers continue to have nipple soreness after two weeks.

Chronic, prolonged sore nipples: If nipple pain extends beyond 2 weeks, assess and treat the condition.

- **Poor positioning of the baby at breast.** Soreness and bruising is likely to be in a crescent shape or "stripes." Correct positioning by assisting the mother to put as much of the areola into the infant's mouth as possible.
- **Tight frenulum (tongue-tie)** that impedes suckling. Severe tightness may be relieved by surgical clipping.
- **Candida infection.** Dark pink, painful areas on breast/nipple. Evidence of thrush in infant. Treatment and use of antifungal medications is discussed on page 23.
- **Bacterial infection.** Complaints of nipple pain with cracks, fissures, ulcers, or exudate. Of these women, there is a 64% chance of having a positive bacterial skin culture.
- Obtain a nipple culture from an unwashed cracked nipple before breastfeeding, using a cotton-tipped culturette.

Medical treatment options for *S. aureus* infection:

- Antibacterial topical ointment to affected area
- Oral antibiotic therapy: penicillinase resistant (dicloxacillin, cephalosporin, erythromycin)
- Nasal mupirocin (Bactroban) ointment may help reduce carrier state.

INTERVENTION OUTCOMES FOR MOTHERS WITH SORE, CRACKED NIPPLES AND S. AUREUS POSITIVE CULTURE

OUTCOME	TEACHING BREASTFEEDING TECHNIQUES	TOPICAL MUPIROCIN	TOPICAL FUSIDIC ACID	ORAL ANTIBIOTICS
Improved	9% (2)	16% (4)	36% (5)	79% (15)
Same	56% (13)	56% (14)	43% (6)	16% (3)
Worse	35% (8)	28% (7)	21% (3)	5% (1)

(Livingston, 1999)

Guidelines for Care

- Use breast shell sore nipple inserts which protects the nipple/areola tissue. Air holes provide air circulation for healing. Ointments can be applied before putting on the shell.
- Apply moist heat to affected breast before each feeding.
- Offer the least sore breast first.
- Make sure the infant is effectively positioned on the breast.
- Alternate position of the infant at each feeding.
- Give ibuprofen (Motrin) or acetaminophen (Tylenol) for pain, if needed.
- Make sure the mother is not using plastic liners on bras and pads.
- Use a fresh breast pad after each feeding.
- Use warm water or purified lanolin or topical antibiotic on sore areas of nipples.
- Avoid using drying agents such as soap or alcohol on the nipple area.
- Avoid removal of all the ointment/cream before the baby breastfeeds. Ointments, creams are not absorbed through the mucous membranes.
- Suggest temporary expression or pumping if the mother is in such extreme pain that she cannot breastfeed. Remove breastmilk as often as the infant would feed to avoid engorgement.

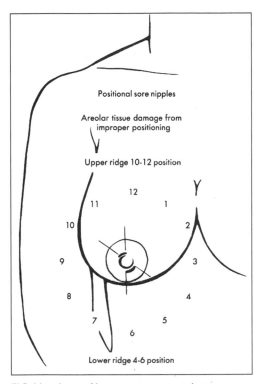

Positional sore nipples

Areolar tissue damage from improper positioning

Upper ridge 10-12 position

12

11   1

10   2

9   3

8   4

7   5

6

Lower ridge 4-6 position

FIG 11 Area of breast soreness and trauma, as related to a clock face. *Imagine the face of a clock superimposed on right breast. Soreness usually develops in the crescent around the perimeter of the nipple at 10 to 12 o'clock position and below the perimeter of the nipple at 4 to 6 o'clock position. With the left breast, maximal potential for soreness is, similarly, at 12 to 2 o'clock and 6 to 8 o'clock positions.*

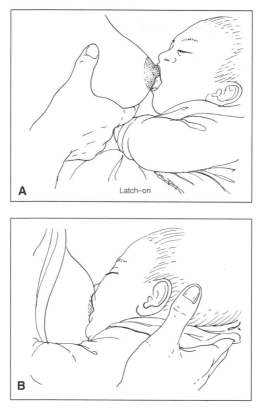

FIG 12 Latch-on *A. Mouth gaped open.*
B. Grasping breast.

Nipples, Inverted

General information:

True inverted nipples are uncommon. If inversion is identified during pregnancy, the mother can anticipate that she may need special interventions in order to breastfeed; therefore prenatal nipple assessment is essential. (See color plates 30 and 31 in *Clinical lactation: A visual guide*.)

Guidelines for Care

Assess the nipple for protractability to see if the inversion is simple or complete. If simple, manual pressure behind the nipple often moves it outward to protract. If complete, the nipple may not respond to manual pressure and remains inverted until the infant goes to breast (see FIG 2 on page 4).

Simple inversion:

- Just before the feeding, use manual pressure or suction* to draw out the nipple for the infant to grasp. While the nipple is still everted, the mother puts the baby to breast.
- Generally, after several weeks of breastfeeding, the nipple everts easily (form follows function) and this pre-feeding maneuver may no longer be necessary.
- Consider using a nipple shield temporarily to get the infant on the breast. Later, the infant can be weaned away from the nipple shield by gradually reducing its use.
- Avoid using breast shells, as they have not been shown to be an effective treatment for inversion.
- Remind the mother that how the nipple looks when the baby is not breastfeeding may not mimic its shape or form in the baby's mouth. The negative pressure

exerted by a vigorously suckling infant usually is sufficient to obtain milk, even from a fully inverted nipple.

Complete or true inversion: If the infant is unable to grasp the nipple to feed, the mother may pump milk from the completely inverted nipple to maintain comfort and use for supplementary feeds. If the infant can feed from her other breast, the mother has options to:

- Continue removing milk from the inverted nipple by pumping or hand expression and breastfeed on the opposite breast.
- Stop pumping or removing milk from the inverted side (involute the breast) and breastfeed from one side only. Reassure that many mothers breastfeed from one side only and their babies grow well.

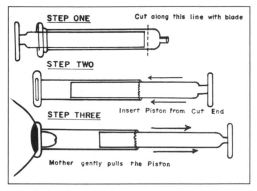

FIG 13-A Disposable syringe device.

*Remove the protrusion on the needle end of a 10 cc
disposable plastic syringe by cutting it with a sharp
blade 1 cm from the nozzle. Remove the piston and
place it in the cut end of the syringe barrel since the
cut edges may be ragged. This is an inexpensive homemade device to create nipple suction (Kesaree et al.
1993).*

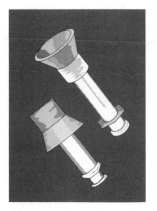

FIG 13-B Commercial nipple suction device
provides gentle suction to evert nipple.

Plugged Ducts

A plugged duct is a tender linear area over a breast duct or painful lump in the lactating breast. It can be caused by skipped or delayed feeding, pressure from tight clothing or bra, sleeping in a position that puts pressure on one area of the breast, or breastfeeding from one side only. If the plugged duct is not treated, it can lead to a breast infection.

Guidelines for Care

- Gently massage 3–4 times a day above and around, but not directly on, the tender area of the breast.
- Breastfeed first on the breast that has the plugged duct.
- Apply moist heat 3–5 minutes before a feeding.
- Change the position of the infant at each feeding to allow more complete emptying of the ducts.
- Check to see if the nursing bra or outer clothing is too tight, causing pressure.

Premature Infant, Discharge Instructions

- Plan to have household help and to spend the first week or two concentrating on the baby. Limit visitors.
- Eat well (fruits and vegetables), drink plenty of water. Sleep when the baby sleeps.
- Calculate the 24-hour minimum caloric needs of the infant before hospital discharge, based on the baby's weight on discharge day.
- Pump 3 times a day to maintain an extra milk supply until the infant is over 6 pounds.
- Supplement with expressed breastmilk or formula if a third of the caloric requirement is not being met by exclusive breastfeeding (about every 8 hours).
- Take plenty of time for feedings at the breast. Watch for signs of infant stress or overstimulation during feedings such as clenched fist with white knuckles, fingers splayed out wide, cheeks and chin sagging, furrowed brow, arm bent at elbow with raised hand (stop sign), legs up as if in a leg lift, arching away, averting gaze by turning head away, yawns, hiccups. Let the baby rest when these cues occur.
- Breastfeed the infant every 3 hours, weighing before and after feedings; note the 24 hours minimum intake necessary as calculated by the care-provider.
- Breastfeed "on cue." If infant acts hungry before 3 hours, go ahead and nurse.
- Keep a record of the number of wet diapers and stools baby has each day.

Look for signs the preemie is getting enough:
- At least 6–9 wet cloth diapers (5–6 disposable diapers) every 24 hours. Urine should be pale in color and mild smelling.

- At least 2–5 good-sized bowel movements every 24 hours during the first 6 weeks.
- A weight gain of at least 4–5 ounces a week. (Use similar weight clothing when baby is weighed). Measure the amount of milk the baby takes at the breast by weighing baby before and after feeding. Record the difference (see Weight Checks).

Supplementation

General information:

Supplementation requires consideration of (1) the fluid and (2) the container that will be used to supplement human milk feedings.

Guidelines for Care

Supplemental fluids should be one of the following, beginning with the optimal choice first:

- mother's own fresh raw milk
- mother's own refrigerated milk
- mother's own frozen milk
- artificial baby milk

General Instructions for Supplementation

All devices discussed should be used with the infant held in arms semi-upright. Particularly with containers where milk flow can overwhelm the baby's ability to manage it, the baby should not be propped in an infant seat or lying down. To cue the infant, gently brush her lower lip with the device containing milk. Wait for her mouth to open widely and her tongue to protrude and form a trough, thus "inviting" the container to provide fluid.

Syringe: A 30 ml barrel is convenient to use and requires only one or two syringes per feeding, as each can be quickly refilled. Draw the milk into the barrel and introduce a small bolus into the corner of the infant's mouth, aimed at the inner cheek surface to reduce the likelihood of choking. If the plunger is removed, the baby's own suckling will often draw fluid into the mouth without difficulty.

Spoon or medicine spoon: Use a standard household spoon with a capacity of about 5 ml. When the infant's mouth is open and her tongue is

121

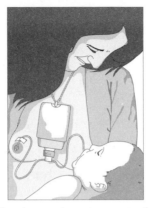

FIG 14   Supplemental nursing system feeding
tube device.

troughed, tip a small bolus of milk into the
trough. Wait for her to swallow and repeat the
process. In very young newborns and premature infants, the baby may lap fluid from the
spoon before sipping.

Cup: A small container, such as a shot glass or
2-dram medicine cup that tapers from a wider
rim to a narrower base works well. Use as described for a spoon (above).

Tube Feeding Device: A device that feeds milk to
the baby through narrow, flexible tubing can be
purchased commercially or made using about
18–24 inches of a small-diameter French tubing
and a container of milk. One end of the tube
terminates in the milk source, and the other is
placed on the pad of the feeder's finger, usually
the index finger but sometimes the thumb.
Elicit a feeding response from the baby as described previously, then gently introduce the

finger (with the tube on it) into the infant's mouth. Slide the finger gently into the baby's mouth and nestle the fleshy finger pad to the roof of the infant's mouth near the juncture of the hard and soft palate; the tube will lie between the finger pad and the roof of the infant's mouth. Sucking motions of the infant's tongue will siphon milk through the tubing at a rate controlled by the baby.

If the tube feeding device is taped to the breast, it should terminate flush with the end of the mother's nipple. This will prevent the baby from sucking only on the tube and provide stimulation to the breast for milk production. When supplemented in this manner, the baby's nutritional integrity is protected even as an inadequate, or not yet established, milk supply can be stimulated.

Surgery, Infant

General information:

Breastfeeding as long as possible before surgery and as quickly as possible following the procedure reduces trauma for the child and the mother. Preparing the breastfeeding infant or child for surgery is similar to preparing the non-breastfed child.

Guidelines for Care

- The infant may breastfeed up to 2 hours prior to the induction of anesthesia. Breastmilk is considered a clear fluid.
- Except for bowel surgeries, young infants can safely breastfeed as soon as they wake from anesthesia.
- Assist the mother to pump her milk if the child is not able to breastfeed beyond 4–6 hours post surgery.

Surgery, Maternal

General information:

Fortunately a breastfeeding mother who must undergo a surgical procedure is more likely to be treated as an outpatient rather than be hospitalized. As a result, separation because of hospitalization is not as frequent a problem for the breastfeeding couple as it was a few years ago. Most concerns center on the transfer of anesthesia and analgesics into breastmilk.

Guidelines for Care

- Before mother goes to surgery, pump and store enough milk so that at least 2 feedings can be given postoperatively, if necessary.
- Provide breast pump for pumping milk for 4 hours postsurgery.
- Resume breastfeeding infant after 4 hours postsurgery.

DRUG	PEAK MILK CONCENTRATION	COMMENTS
Thiopental	At 2 hrs = 0.9 µg/mL	Used to induce general anesthesia. Transfer to infant is inconsequential.
Propofol	0.7 µg/mL	Used to induce general anesthesia. Rapid clearance.
Fentanyl	Within 1 hr = 0.4 ng/mL Adult half-life: 3–4 hrs. Newborn half-life: 3–13 hrs.	Rapid clearance. Not detectable in breastmilk 4–7 hrs. after administration.
Meperidine (Demoral)	500 ng/mL	Infant neurobehavioral depression is possible.
Morphine	60 ng/mL	Multiple doses may cause infant sedation and ineffective suckling.
Midazolam (Versed)	9 ng/mL	Low passage rate into breastmilk. Not detected at 7 hrs. No apparent effect on breastfed infants.

Twins, Breastfeeding

General information:

Breastfeeding more than one infant at a time is entirely possible. The ease of doing so depends on the mother's motivation to breastfeed, her social support and, possibly, her organizational skills. The same basic breastfeeding principles that apply to a singleton also apply to twins. While mothers may often find that simultaneous breastfeeding is most easily accomplished and appreciated when the babies are small and feeding frequently, many mothers of multiples find it important to breastfeed the babies separately as they get larger and/or as their own needs become more individualized.

Guidelines for Care (for term or near-term twins, triplets, quads, quints)

Advise the mother to:

- Begin feedings as soon after birth as possible. Following a Cesarean birth, the time of the first feedings will vary according to the mother's condition.
- Feed both babies simultaneously to save time. This works especially well when the babies are small and tend to feed at the same time. Later the infants may be fed separately to meet their individual hunger and nurturance needs.
- Use several *firm* pillows to support the infants during feedings. We recommend a pillow especially made to assist mothers of twins.
- Switch breasts for feedings so that each infant feeds on both sides to balance individual milk needs and enhance the infants' need for visual exercise. Because babies do not always have similar feeding

styles, both breasts should be offered to each baby to optimize adequate milk transfer.

- Eat frequent snacks of nutritious, high-calorie "fast foods" (cheese and crackers, cut-up vegetables, yogurt, peanut butter, fruit, ice cream). The mother of multiples may be at risk for nutritional depletion.
- Insist on household and infant care help from family members or, if possible, professional house cleaners.
- Accommodate for individual differences in eating, sleeping, and elimination patterns between infants even though they may be identical genetically.

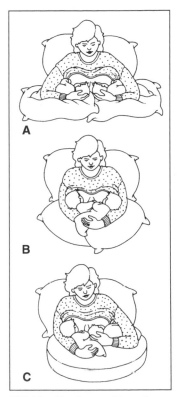

FIG 15   Feeding positions for
twins: (A) Football, (B) Cross,
and (C) Mixed. (Drawing by Ruth
Linstromberg.)

Weight Checks

- Weigh the infant with an electronic scale. Portable electronic scales are available.
- Encourage the mother to think of the scale as a short-term aid in caring for the baby.
- Calibrate the scale to register 0. Weight can be measured in both pounds and ounces or in grams.
- Before and after feeds to measure intake: Weigh the baby before a feed and after the feed. Subtract the pre-feed weight from post-feed weight. The baby can be weighed with his clothes on as long as he is wearing the same clothes for both weight measurements.
- Weight gain check: Check weight gain on the same day each week. Remove infant's clothing and place on top of clean light blanket placed on scale.
- The baby's weight can be graphed so that the parents can see the progress in weight gain.
- Weekly weight gains may not be fully accurate due to difference that can occur if the infant has stooled and/or urinated just before the weight check.
- Teach the mother about other measures of intake that she will use when she has returned the scale: the number of wet and "dirty" diapers, and the baby growing out of clothes that previously fit with room to spare.

References

Except for the references listed below, most information in this text is from Riordan and Auerbach, *Breastfeeding and Human Lactation,* 2nd edition, Sudbury, MA: Jones and Bartlett Publisher, 1999. References to color plates are from Auerbach and Riordan, *Clinical lactation: A visual guide.* Sudbury, MA: Jones and Bartlett Publisher, 2000. All materials have been reprinted or adapted with permission.

Breast Assessment

Farina, MA, Newby, BG, and Alani HM: *Innervation of the nipple-areola complex. Plast. Reconstr Surg.* 66:497, 1980.

Breast, creams and gels

Brent, N et al: Sore nipples in breast-feeding women. *Archives of Pediatrics & Adolescent Medicine* 1:1077, 1998.

Buchko BL, et al: Comfort measures in breastfeeding, primiparous women. *JOGNN* 23:46–52, 1993.

Lavergne NA: Does application of tea bags to sore nipples while breastfeeding provide effective relief? *JOGNN* 26:53–58, 1997.

Breast, eczema, impetigo, psoriasis

Amir L: Eczema of the nipple and breast: a case report. *J Hum Lact* 98:173–75, 1993.

Huggins K, Billon SF: Twenty cases of persistent sore nipples: collaboration between lactation consultant and dermatologist. *J Hum Lact* 9:155–60, 1993.

Livingstone V: The treatment of *Staphylococcus Aureus* infected sore nipples: A randomized comparative study. *J Hum Lact* 241–46, 1999.

Breast, hypoplasia

Huggins KE, Petok ES, Mireles O: Markers of lactation insufficiency: a study of 34 mothers. *Current Issues in Clinical Lactation*. Sudbury, MA: Jones and Bartlett Publ. 2000.

Breast, lump

Scott-Conner CE, Schorr SJ: The diagnosis and management of breast problems during pregnancy and lactation. *Am J Surgery* 170:401–4, 1995.

Slavin JL, Billson VR, Oster AG: Nodular breast lesions during pregnancy and lactation. *Histopathology* 22:85, 1993.

Breast, mammaplasty

Higgins S, Haffty BF: Pregnancy and lactation after breast-conserving therapy for early stage breast cancer. *Cancer* 73:2175–180, 1994.

Hurst NM: Lactation after augmentation mammoplasty. *Obstet & Gynecol* 87:30–34, 1996.

Marshall DR, Callan PP, Nicholson W: Breastfeeding after reduction mammaplasty. *Br J Plast Surg* 47:167–79, 1994.

Widdice L: The effects of breast reduction and breast augmentation surgery on lactation: an annotated bibliography. *J Hum Lact* 9:161–67, 1993.

Breast, pain

Heads J, Higgins LC: Perceptions and correlates of nipple pain. *Breastfeed Rev* 3:59–64, 1995.

Mohrbacher N, Stock J: *The breastfeeding answer book* (rev ed). Schaumburg, IL: La Leche League, International, 1997, pp 428–32.

Breast, preference

Mohrbacher N, Stock J: *The breastfeeding answer book* (rev ed). Schaumburg, IL: La Leche League, International, 1997, pp 106–9.

Breast, pumps

Mohrbacher N, Stock J: *The breastfeeding answer book* (rev ed). Schaumburg, IL: La Leche League, International, 1997, pp 546–61.

Auerbach KG: Sequential and simultaneous breast pumping: a comparison. *Int J Nurs Stud* 27:257–65, 1990.

Breast, refusal

Newman J, Wilmott B: Breast rejection: a little-appreciated cause of lactation failure. *Can Fam Phys* 36:449–53, 1990.

Breastmilk, collection and storage

Arnold LDW: Storage containers for human milk: an issue revisited. *J Hum Lact* 11:325–8, 1995.

Mohrbacher N, Stock, J: *The breastfeeding answer book* (rev ed). Schaumburg, IL: La Leche League, International, 1997, pp 487–91.

Pardou A, et al: Human milk banking: influence of storage processes and of bacterial contamination on some milk constituents. *Bio. Neonate* 65:302–9, 1994.

Williamson MT, Murti PK: Effect of storage, time, temperature and composition of containers on biologic components of human milk. *J Hum Lact* 12:31–35, 1996.

Candida/Thrush

Amir, LH: Candida and the lactating breast: predisposing factors. *J Hum Lact* 7:177–81, 1991.

Hancock KF, Spangler AK: There's fungus among us! *J Hum Lact* 9:179–80, 1993.

Johnstone HA, Marcinak JF: Candidiasis in the breastfeeding mother and infant. *JOGNN* 19:171–73, 1990.

Tanguay KE, McBean MR, Jain E: Nipple candidiasis among breastfeeding mothers. *Can Fam Physician* 40:1407–13, 1994.

Cesarean Birth

Kearney MH, Cronenwett LR, Reinhardt R: Cesarean delivery and breastfeeding outcomes. *Birth* 17:97–103, 1990.

Rajan L: The impact of obstetric procedures and analgesia/anesthesia during labour and delivery on breastfeeding. *Midwifery* 10:87–103, 1994.

Chickenpox

Lawrence RA: A review of medical benefits and contraindications to breastfeeding in the United States (Maternal and Child Health Technical Information Bulletin). Arlington, VA: National Center for Education in Maternal and Child Health, 1997.

Peter G, et al eds: *1994 Red Book: American Academy of Pediatrics: Report of the Committee on Infectious Diseases,* 23rd ed. Elk Grove Village, IL: American Academy of Pediatrics, 1994.

Yoshida M, et al: Case report: detection of varicella-zoster virus DNA in maternal breast milk. *J Med Virol* 38:108–9, 1992.

Contraception

Hatcher RA, et al: *Managing contraception.* Tiger, GA: Bridging the Gap Foundation, 1999.

Labbok MH, Howie, PW: Overview and summary: the interface of breastfeeding, natural family planning, and lactational amenorrhea. *Am J Obstet Gynecol* 165:2013–14, 1991.

World Health Organization. WHO: Taskforce on postovulatory methods of fertility regulation. *Lancet* Aug 8, 1998.

Saaikoski, S: Contraception during lactation. *Ann Med* 25:181–4, 1993.

Cytomegalovirus (CMV)

Lawrence RA: A review of medical benefits and contraindications to breastfeeding in the United States. *Maternal and Child Health Technical Information Bulletin.* Arlington, VA: National Center for Education in Maternal and Child Health, 1997.

Minamishima I, et al: Role of breast milk in acquisition of cytomegalovirus infection. *Microbio Immunol* 38:549–52, 1994.

Peter G, et al eds: *1994 Red Book: American Academy of Pediatrics: Report of the Committee on Infectious*

Diseases, 23rd ed. Elk Grove Village, IL: American Academy of Pediatrics, 1994.

Depression, postpartum

Beck CT: Screening methods for postpartum depression. *JOGNN* 24:308–12, 1995.

Cooper PJ, Murray L, Stein A: Psychosocial factors associated with the early termination of breast-feeding. *J Psychosom Res* 37:171–76, 1993.

Hale T: *Clinical therapy in breastfeeding patients.* Amarillo TX: Pharmasoft Medical Publishing, 1999.

Employment

Auerbach KG: Assisting the employed breastfeeding mother. *J Nurse Midwif* 35:26–34, 1990.

Bocar DL: Combining breastfeeding and employment: increasing success. *J. Perinatal & Neonatal Nursing* 11:23, 1997.

Corbett-Dick P, Bezedk SK: Breastfeeding promotion for the employed mother. *J Pediatr Health Care* 11:12–19, 1997.

Hills-Bonczyk SG, et al: Women's experiences with combining breast-feeding and employment. *J Nurs Midwif* 38:257–66, 1993.

Thompson PE, Bell P: Breast-feeding in the workplace: how to succeed. *Iss Comp Pediatr Nurse* 20:1–9, 1997.

Engorgement, breast

Hill PD, Humenick SS: The occurrence of breast engorgement. *J Hum Lact* 10:79–86, 1994.

Humenick SS, Hill PD, Anderson MA: Breast engorgement: patterns and selected outcomes. *J Hum Lact* 10:87–93, 1994.

Moon JL, Humenick SS: Breast engorgement: contributing variables and variables amenable to nursing intervention. *JOGNN* 18:309–15, 1989.

Roberts KL: A comparison of chilled cabbage leaves and chilled gelpaks in reducing breast engorgement. *J Hum Lact* 11:17–20, 1995.

Finger Feeding

Walker M: *Breastfeeding Premature Babies* (unit 14). La Leche League, International, Lactation Consultant Series, New York. Garden City Park: Avery Publishing Group, Inc, 1991.

Formula and Non-Human Milk Feedings

Biancuzzo M: *Breastfeeding the newborn.* St. Louis: Mosby, 1999, p 348–63.

Wink D: Getting through the maze of infant formulas. *AJN* 85:388–92, 1985.

Galactologues

Gupta AP, Gupta PK: Metoclopramide as a lactogogue. *Clin Pediatr* 24:269–72, 1985.

Hale T: *Clinical therapy in breastfeeding patients.* Amarillo, TX: Pharmasoft Medical Publishing, 1999.

Kauppila A, et al.: A dose response relation between improved lactation and metoclopramide. *Lancet* 1(8231):1175–1177, 1983.

Ylikorkal O, et al: Treatment of inadequate lactation. *Br. Med J* 285:249–251, 1982.

Hepatitis B, Hepatitis C

American Academy of Pediatrics Committee on Infectious Diseases: Hepatitis C virus infection. *Pediatrics* 101:481, 1998.

American Academy of Pediatrics: *1997 Red Book: Report of the Committee on Infectious Diseases,* 24th ed., 1997, p 73–79.

Kurauchi O, Furni T, Hakura A, Ishiko H, Sugiyama M, Ohno Y, et al.: Studies on transmission of hepatitis C virus from mother-to-child in the perinatal period. *Arch Gynecol Obstet* 2563:121–26, 1993.

Ho-Hsiung L et al: Absence of infection in breast-fed infants born to hepatitis C virus-infected mothers. *J Pediatrics* 125(4): 589–91, 1995.

Peter G, et al eds: *1994 Red Book: Report of the Committee on Infectious Diseases.* 23rd ed. Elk Grove

Village, IL, American Academy of Pediatrics, 1994, 224–38.

Ruff AJ: Breastmilk, breastfeeding and transmission of viruses to the neonate. *Seminars in Perinatology* 18:510–16, 1994.

Taddio A, Klein J, Koren G: Acyclovir excretion in human breast milk. *Ann Pharmacother* 28:585–86, 1994.

Tseng RYM, Lam CWK, & Tam J: Breastfeeding babies of HBsAg-positive mothers. *Lancet* 2(8618):1032, 1988.

HIV/AIDS

American Academy of Pediatrics, Committee on Pediatric AIDS: Human milk, breastfeeding, and transmission of human immunodeficiency virus in the United States. *Pediatrics* 96:977–79, 1992.

Duprat C, et al: Human immunodeficiency virus type 1 IgA antibody in breast milk and serum. *Pediatr Infect Dis J* 13:603–8, 1994.

Lindberg CE: Perinatal transmission of HIV: how to counsel women. *Maternal Child Nurs J* 20:207–12, 1995.

Van de Perre P: Postnatal transmission of human immunodeficiency virus type 1: the breast-feeding dilemma. *Am J Obstet Gynecol* 173:483–87, 1995.

Hindmilk, feedings

Meier P: Expressing hindmilk for baby. *Special care Nursery.* Chicago: Rush-Presbyterian-St Luke's Medical Center, 1996.

Valentine CJ, Hurst NM, Schandler RJ: Hindmilk improves weight gain in low-birth-weight infants fed human milk. *J Pediatr Gastroenterol* 18:474–77, 1994.

Immunizations

Chirico G, et al: Hepatitis B immunization in infants of hepatitis B surface antigen-negative mothers. *Pediatrics* 92:717–79, 1993.

Hahn-Zoric M, et al: Antibody responses to parenteral and oral vaccines are impaired by conventional and low protein formulas as compared to breast-feeding. *Acta Paediatr Scand* 1137–42, 1990.

Lawrence R: *Breastfeeding: A guide for the medical profession,* 5th ed. St. Louis: Mosby, 1999.

Pabst J, Spady D: Effect of breast-feeding on antibody response to conjugate vaccine. *Lancet* 336:269–70, 1990.

Centers for Disease Control: General recommendations on immunization. *MMRW* 43(RR-1):1–38, 1994.

Inadequate milk supply, actual
Neifert MR, Seacat, JM: Lactation insufficiency: a rational approach. *Birth* 14:182–88, 1987.

Motil KG, Sheng HP, Montandon CM: Case report: failure to thrive in a breastfed infant is associated with maternal dietary protein and energy restriction. *J Am Coll Nutr* 13:203–8, 1994.

Powers NG: Slow weight gain and low milk supply in the breastfeeding dyad. Clinical Aspects of Human Milk and Lactation. *Clinics in Perinatology* 26:399–429, 1999.

Willis CE, Livingstone V: Infant insufficient milk syndrome associated with maternal postpartum hemorrhage. *J Hum Lact* 11:123–26, 1995.

Inadequate milk supply, perceived
Hill PD, Aldag JC: Insufficient milk supply among black and white breast-feeding mothers. *Res Nurs Health* 16:203–11, 1993.

Induced lactation
Nemba K: Induced lactation: a study of 37 non-puerperal mothers. *J Trop Pediatr* 40:240–2, 1994.

Infant, insufficient weight gain
Dewey KG, et al: Growth of breast-fed infants deviates from current reference data: a pooled analy-

sis of US, Canadian and European data sets. *Pediatrics* 96:495–503, 1995.

Meier P, et al: A new scale for in-home test-weighing for mothers of preterm and high risk infants. *J. Hum Lact 10:*163–68, 1994.

Jaundice

James JM, Williams SD, Osborn LM: Discontinuation of breast-feeding infrequent among jaundiced neonates treated at home. *Pediatrics* 92:153–55, 1993.

Madlin-Kay DJ: Evaluation and management of newborn jaundice by Midwest family physicians. *J. Family Practice* 47:461, 1998.

Martinez JC, et al: Hyperbilirubinemia in the breast-fed newborn: a controlled trial of four interventions. *Pediatrics* 91:470–3, 1993.

Newman TB, Maisels MJ: Evaluation and treatment of jaundice in the term newborn: a kinder, gentler approach. *Pediatrics* 89:809–18, 1992.

Mastitis

Bevin TH, Persok CK: Breastfeeding difficulties and a breast abscess associated with a galactocele: a case report. *J Hum Lact* 9:177–78, 1993.

Dixon JM: Breast infection. *Br Med J* 309:946–49, 1994.

Fetherston C: Risk factors for lactation mastitis. *J Hum Lact* 14:101–9, 1998.

Foxman B, Schwartz K, Looman SJ: Breastfeeding practices and lactation mastitis. *Soc Sci Med* 38:755–61, 1994.

Mohrbacher N, Stock J: *The breastfeeding answer book* (rev ed). Schaumburg, IL: La Leche League, International, 1997, pp 418–26.

Riordan J, Nichols F: A descriptive study of lactation mastitis in long-term breastfeeding women. *J Hum Lact* 6:53–8, 1990.

Medications, maternal

American Academy of Pediatrics Committee on Drugs: Transfer of drugs and other chemicals into human milk. *Pediatrics* 93:137–50, 1994.

Briggs GC, et al: *Drugs in pregnancy and lactation,* (5th ed). Baltimore: Williams & Wilkins, 1998.

Hale T: *Clinical therapy in breastfeeding patients.* Amarillo TX: Pharmasoft Medical Publishing, 1999.

Hale T: *Medications and mothers' milk,* 8th ed. Amarillo TX: Pharmasoft Medical Publishing, 1999.

Ito S, et al: Prospective follow-up of adverse reactions in breast-fed infants exposed to maternal medication. *Am J Obstet Gynecol* 168:1393–1399, 1993.

Lawrence R: *Breastfeeding: a guide for the medical profession,* 5th ed. St. Louis: Mosby, 1999.

Nipple, blister ("bleb")

Noble R: Milk under the skin (milk blister)–a simple problem causing other breast conditions. *Breastfeeding Review* 2:118–19, 1991.

Nipple, leaking

Mohrbacher N, Stock J: *The breastfeeding answer book* (rev ed). Schaumburg, IL: La Leche League, International, 1997, pp 208–9.

Nipples, sore

Brent N, et al: Sore nipples in breast-feeding women. *Archives of Pediatrics & Adolescent Medicine* 1:1077, 1998.

Foxman B, Schwartz K, Looman SJ: Breastfeeding practices and lactation mastitis. *Soc Sci Med* 38:755–61, 1994.

Huggins KE, Billion SF: Twenty cases of persistent sore nipples: collaboration between lactation consultant and dermatologist. *J Hum Lact* 9:155–60, 1993.

Livingston V: The treatment of staphyloccous aureus in infected sore nipples: A randomized comparative study. *J Hum Lact* 15(3):241–46, 1999.

Nipples, inverted

Alexander JM, Grant AM, Campbell MJ: Randomised controlled trial of breast shells and Hoffmans's exercises for inverted and non-protractile nipples. *BMJ* 304:1030–32, 1992.

Kesaree N, et al: Treatment of inverted nipples using a disposable syringe. *J. Hum Lact* 9:27–29, 1993.

Supplementation

Coates MM, Riordan J: Breastfeeding during maternal or infant illness. *In* Chute GE ed: *NAACOG's Clinical Issues in Perinatal and Women's Health Nursing* 3:683–94, 1992.

Glover J: Supplementation of breastfeeding newborns: a flow chart for decision-making. *J Hum Lact* 11:127–31, 1995.

Mohrbacher N, Stock J: *The breastfeeding answer book* (rev ed). Schaumburg, IL: La Leche League, International, 1997, pp 540–46.

Surgery, infant

Litman RS, Wu CL, Quinlivan JK: Gastric volume and pH in infants fed clear liquids and breast milk prior to surgery. *Anesth Analg,* 79:482–85, 1994.

Nicholson SC, Schreiner MS: Feed the babies. *La Leche League International, Breastfeeding Abstracts* 15(1):3–4, 1995.

Surgery, maternal

Biddle C: When the breast-feeding mother faces surgery. *Contemporary Nurse Practitioner* July/August:15–20, 1995.

Twins, breastfeeding

Biancuzzo M: Breastfeeding preterm twins: a case report. *Birth* 21:96–100, 1994.

Gromada KK: Breastfeeding twins and higher-order multiples. *JOGNN* 27:441–49, 1998.

Mead LJ, et al: Breastfeeding success with preterm quadruplets. *JOGNN* 21:221–27, 1992.

APPENDICES

A. Via Christi Assessment Tool

B. Lactation Web Sites

C. Common Spanish Phrases for Breastfeeding

D. Time line of postpartum events

E. Sample letter to request third-party payment for breast pump

F. Immediate, Postpartum Breastfeeding Decision Tree

G. Conversion Chart of Pounds and Ounces to Grams

H. Patient History

I. Conversion Tables

J. Standardized Height and Weight Growth Charts

Appendix A

VIA CHRISTI BREASTFEEDING ASSESSMENT TOOL

	0	1	2	SCORE
Latch-on	No latch-on achieved	Latch-on after repeated attempts	Eagerly grasped breast to latch on	
Length of time before latch-on and suckle	Over 10 min	4–6 min	0–3 min	
Suckling	Did not suckle	Suckled but needs encouragement	Suckled rhythmically & lips flanged	
Audible Swallowing	None	Only if stimulated	Under 48 hrs: Intermittent Over 48 hrs: frequent	
Mom's Evaluation	Not pleased	Somewhat pleased	Pleased	

TOTAL SCORE _____

The Via Christi Breastfeeding Assessment Tool assigns a score of 0, 1, 2 to five factors. Scores range from 1 to 10.

- 0–3 = High Risk: Close, immediate postdischarge follow-up. Phone call and visit to provider within 3 days. **All mothers who have had breast surgery are considered high risk.**
- 4–6 = Medium Risk: Postdischarge phone call within 5 days. Follow-up as per protocol.
- 7–10 = Low Risk: Info given to mother and routine phone call.

LACTATION WEB SITES

Topic	*Website*
American Academy of Pediatrics Policy Statement on Breastfeeding	http://www.aap.org/policy/re9729.html
American Dietetic Association: Promotion of Breastfeeding site	http://www.eatright.org/adap0697.html
Answers to breastfeeding questions, concerns	http://www.lactationinnovation.com http://www.parentsplace.com/expert/lactation/basics/ http://www.promom.org http://www.rosebaby.com/
Breast pumps and supplies	http://www.breastpumps-etc.com http://www.medela.com/ http://www.hollister.com http://www.lecheleague.org/Catalog/Pump96.html

Breastfeeding information and promotion (slides, photos, video clips, etc.)	http://www.breastfeeding.com
	http://www.infactcanada.ca/index.htm
	http://www.geddespro.com
Parent and staff breastfeeding education (videos, print materials)	http://www.xrsgroup.com
	http://www.injoyvideos.com
	http://www.noodlesoup.com
	http://www.members.aol.com/marshalact/naba
Courses on breastfeeding	http://www.txsu.edu/~wsucofhp/N791/class_materials/
	http://www.breastfeedingbasics.org/
	http://www.members.aol.com/bscenter
	http://www.aboutus.com/a100/healthed/
Drugs and breastfeeding	http://www.prl.humc.edu/obgyn/public/tearatog/riska-c.htm
	http://www.perinatalpub.com
	http://www.monarch-design.com/baby/direc.html

(continued)

Topic	Website
Baby Friendly USA	*http://www.aboutus.com/a100/bfusa*
Human milk banking	*http://www.hmbana.org*
	http://www.nursingmother.com/all_about/all_about/all_about_milk_banks.html
	http://www.mmbaustin.org/
International Board for Lactation Consultant Examiners (registry of lactation consultants examination blueprint)	*http://www.iblce.org*
International Lactation Consultant Association (conferences, membership)	*http://users.erols.com/ilca/ilca.html*
Jones and Bartlett Publishing Company (books on breastfeeding)	*http://www.jbpub.com/*
Journal articles	*http://www.medscape.com/*
	http://www4.ncbi.nlm.nih.gov/PubMed/

148

La Leche League, International (publications, seminars, LLL leaders, answers breastfeeding questions)	*http://www.lalecheleague.org*
Legislation related to breastfeeding	*http://www.lalecheleague.org/LawMain.html*
LACTNET archives (breastfeeding discussion)	*http://peach.ease.lsoft.com/archives/lactnet.html*
Links to other Web sites	*http://www.bflrc.com/links/adx.htm/*
	www.promom.org
Setting up lactation services	*http://www.hsls.com*
WABA (World Alliance for Breastfeeding Action)	*http://www.waba.org.br/*
World Health Organization, AIDS Information	*http://www.unaids.org/highband/document/mother-to-child/index.html*

Appendix C

COMMON SPANISH PHRASES FOR BREASTFEEDING

SPANISH	*ENGLISH*
Leche materna	Breastmilk
Calostro	Colostrum
Madre	Mother
Bebe	Baby
Consultor de lactancia	Lactation consultant
Consejera	Nurse
Masaje del pecho	Breast massage
Expresion manual	Hand expression
No usar chupetes	No pacifiers
No usar biberones	No bottles
Succionar los pechos	Pump breasts
Alimentación suplementaria	Supplemental feeding
Alimentación de pecho	Breastfeeding
Amamantar a su bebe	Breastfeed your baby
Pecho	Breast
Pezón	Nipple
Ya se puede amamantar a su nino(a)	You can breastfeed your baby now
¿Le va bien cuando da pecho?	How is breastfeeding going?
¿Cuantás veces come el niño cada vez que le da el pecho?	How often does the baby breastfeed each day?
¿Cuántos pañales mojados tiene el niño por día?	How many wet diapers does the baby have each day?

151

SPANISH	ENGLISH
¿Está recibiendo suficiente? ¿Cinco a seis pañales mojados por día?	Is he/she getting enough? 5–6 wet diapers each day?
¿Está recibiendo suficiente? ¿Cuatro o más deposiciones por día?	Is he/she getting enough? 4 or more bowel movement a day?
¿Cuántas veces defeca el niño por día?	How many dirty diapers does the baby have each day?
Le da pecho cuando quiera el niño, usualmente ocho a doce veces por día.	Breastfeed as often as the baby wants, usually 8–12 times a day.
Usted puede comer lo que quiera a menos que el niño se ponga malo después de que coma algo en particular.	You can eat what you want unless you notice the baby is fussy after you eat certain foods.
Sus pesones van a ester un poquito enflamados. Pero en unos cuantos días se le va a quitar.	Your nipples may be sore for a few days but it will go away.

Appendix D

Time line of postpartum events

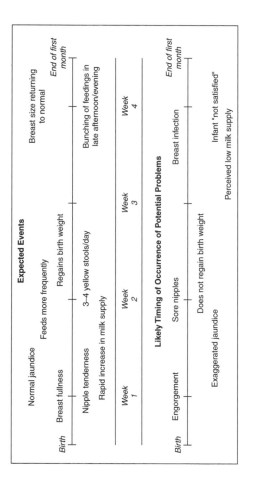

Expected Events

Birth — Week 1 — Week 2 — Week 3 — Week 4 — End of first month

- Normal jaundice
- Feeds more frequently
- Breast size returning to normal
- Breast fullness
- Regains birth weight
- Nipple tenderness
- 3–4 yellow stools/day
- Bunching of feedings in late afternoon/evening
- Rapid increase in milk supply

Likely Timing of Occurrence of Potential Problems

Birth — Week 1 — Week 2 — Week 3 — Week 4 — End of first month

- Engorgement
- Sore nipples
- Breast infection
- Does not regain birth weight
- Infant "not satisfied"
- Exaggerated jaundice
- Perceived low milk supply

Appendix E

Sample letter to request third-party payment for breast pump

Date

Insured:

Policy Number:

Re: Electric Breast Pump Rental

To Whom It May Concern:

Dr. _____, a neonatologist in the Special Care Nursery at Rush-Presbyterian-St. Luke's Medical Center, has prescribed human milk feedings for _____, who was born on _____, and whose parents are _____. Because this infant is too small and/or ill to feed at the breast, the mother must remove her milk with an electric breast pump, store it, and transport it to the Special Care Nursery so that it can be fed to her infant using a gavage tube.

A hospital grade electric breast pump with a double collection kit is necessary for extracting milk under these circumstances. Randomized controlled trials have shown that manual and/or battery-operated pumps, intended for occasional use by mothers of healthy infants, are inadequate for mothers who must initiate and maintain lactation in the absence of a nursing infant. Although hospital grade electric pumps can be purchased (approximately $900), they are more economical to rent on a short-term basis. We estimate that this mother will require use of the pump for approximately _____.

I trust that this information will expedite insurance coverage of the electric pump rental for this mother and infant. Should there be additional questions, please contact me at the above address/telephone.

Sincerely,

Paula P. Meier, RN, DNSc, FAAN
NICU Lactation Program Director

Appendix F

Immediate Postpartum Breastfeeding Decision Tree

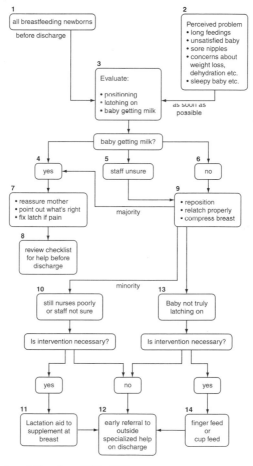

from J Hum Lact 12(2), 1996

CONVERSION CHART OF POUNDS AND OUNCES TO GRAMS

Pounds		*Ounces*														
	0	1	2	3	4	5	6	7	8	9	10	11	12	13	14	15
0	—	28	57	85	113	142	170	198	227	255	283	312	430	369	397	425
1	454	482	510	539	567	595	624	652	680	709	737	765	794	822	850	879
2	907	936	964	992	1021	1049	1077	1106	1134	1162	1191	1219	1247	1276	1304	1332
3	1361	1389	1417	1446	1474	1503	1531	1559	1588	1616	1644	1673	1701	1729	1758	1786
4	1814	1843	1871	1899	1928	1956	1984	2013	2041	2070	2098	2126	2155	2183	2211	2240
5	2268	2296	2325	2353	2381	2410	2438	2466	2495	2523	2551	2580	2608	2637	2665	2693
6	2722	2750	2778	2807	2835	2863	2893	2920	2948	2977	3005	3033	3062	3090	3118	3137
7	3175	3203	3232	3260	3289	3317	3345	3374	3402	3430	3459	3487	3515	3544	3572	3600

8	3629	3657	3685	3714	3742	3770	3799	3827	3856	3884	3912	3941	3969	3997	4026	4054
9	4082	4111	4139	4167	4196	4224	4252	4281	4309	4337	4366	4394	4423	4451	4479	4508
10	4536	4564	4593	4621	4649	4678	4706	4734	4763	4719	4819	4848	4876	4904	4933	4961
11	4990	5018	5046	5075	5103	3131	5160	5188	5216	5245	5273	5301	5330	5358	5386	5415
12	5443	5471	5500	5528	5557	5585	5613	5642	5670	5698	5727	5755	5783	5812	5840	5868
13	5897	5925	5953	5982	6010	6038	6067	6095	6123	6152	6180	6209	6237	6265	6294	6322
14	6350	6379	6407	6435	6464	6492	6520	6549	6577	6605	6634	6662	6690	6719	6747	6776
15	6804	6832	6860	6889	6917	6945	6973	7002	7030	7059	7087	7115	7144	7172	7201	7228

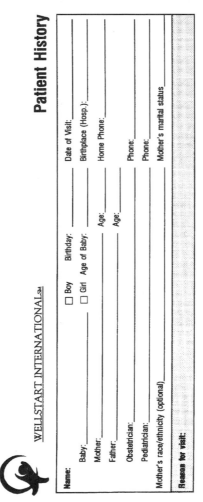

WELLSTART INTERNATIONAL℠

Patient History

Name:

Baby: ☐ Boy Birthday: _____ Date of Visit: _____
       ☐ Girl Age of Baby: _____ Birthplace (Hosp.): _____

Mother: _____ Age: _____ Home Phone: _____

Father: _____ Age: _____

Obstetrician: _____ Phone: _____

Pediatrician: _____ Phone: _____

Mother's race/ethnicity (optional) _____ Mother's marital status

Reason for visit:

MATERNAL HISTORY

1. Are you allergic to any medication? ☐ Yes ☐ No If yes, please list: _____

2. Have you ever had any of the following? Please check (✔) all that apply.

☐ Abnormal pap smear
☐ Allergy/asthma
☐ Anemia
☐ Cancer
☐ Constipation/hemorrhoids
☐ Depression/blues

☐ Diabetes
☐ Diarrhea (chronic)
☐ Heart disease
☐ High blood pressure
☐ Infertility
☐ Kidney disease/bladder
   infection

☐ Liver disease/hepatitis
☐ Thyroid disorders
☐ Tuberculosis
☐ Venereal disease
☐ None known
☐ Other: _____

3. Have you ever had any of the following problems or procedures related to your breasts? Please check (✔) all that apply.

☐ Biopsy
☐ Lumps

☐ Nipple problems:
☐ Surgery: _____
☐ None

159

4. Are you taking the following medications? Please check (✔) all that apply.
   - ☐ Prenatal vitamin-mineral
   - ☐ Other vitamins
   - ☐ Iron
   - ☐ Other minerals
   - ☐ Diet pills
   - ☐ Antihistamines/cold remedies
   - ☐ Laxatives/antacids
   - ☐ Diuretics/water pills
   - ☐ Aspirin/pain pills
   - ☐ Birth control pills
   - ☐ Antibiotics
   - ☐ None of the above
   - ☐ Other drugs_____

PERINATAL HISTORY   List all pregnancies:

5.

Date Preg. Ended	Weeks Gesta- tion	Sex	Birth Weight	Complications of Pregnancy	Complications of Labor and Delivery	*Type of Anes- thesia	Type of Delivery		Breast- feeding Duration
							Vag.	C/S	

*Anesthesia: ① None   ② Local   ③ Epidural   ④ Spinal   ⑤ General (asleep)
              ⑥ Other_____

160

6. Did you have any of the following during this pregnancy? Please check (✓) all that apply.

☐ Anemia (low iron level)
☐ Fever
☐ Gestational diabetes
☐ High blood pressure
☐ Nausea/vomiting (severe)
☐ Premature labor
☐ Urinary tract infection
☐ Medication
☐ None of the above
☐ Other:_____

7. Did you have any of the following during this labor and delivery? Please check (✓) all that apply.

☐ Drugs to induce or speed labor. If yes, for how long during labor was this drug administered? _____ hours
☐ Premature rupture of membranes
☐ Drugs to control high blood pressure
☐ Drugs to control pain
☐ Fever
☐ Antibiotics
☐ Hemorrhage
☐ None of the above
☐ Other:_____

8. With this labor and delivery, did you have any of the following? Please check (✓) all that apply.

☐ Total labor longer than 30 hours
☐ Pushing stage longer than 2 hours
☐ Episiotomy or vaginal tear
☐ Tear that involved the rectum (a "third or fourth degree" laceration)
☐ Breech presentation
☐ Forceps delivery
☐ Vacuum extraction
☐ None of the above

9. How would you rate your labor and delivery experience? Please check (✓) all that apply.
   - ☐ Easy
   - ☐ Difficult
   - ☐ Painful
   - ☐ Long
   - ☐ Short
   - ☐ Average length
   - ☐ Just what I'd expected
   - ☐ Not what I'd expected
   - ☐ Other_____

10. Postpartum complications? Please check (✓) all that apply.
   - ☐ Urinary/other infection
   - ☐ Excessive bleeding (hemorrhage)
   - ☐ High blood pressure
   - ☐ Low blood pressure (shock)
   - ☐ None of the above
   - ☐ Other_____

11. Did the baby have any of the following shortly after birth? Please check (✓) all that apply.
   - ☐ Breathing problems
   - ☐ Fever
   - ☐ High hematocrit
   - ☐ Jaundice
   - ☐ Low blood sugar
   - ☐ Meconium aspiration
   - ☐ None of the above

   - ☐ Medications:_____
   - ☐ Other:_____

12. How soon after delivery did you first put your baby to your breast?_____

13. Were you and your baby separated for more than 2 hours while in the hospital?   ☐ Yes   ☐ No

14. While in the hospital, how many times in 24 hours did you breastfeed your baby?
   ☐ Less than 8 times   ☐ 8-12 times (every 2-3 hours)   ☐ More than 12 times

15. While in the hospital, what was the longest time between breastfeeding?   Day:_____   Night:_____

16. Did you have any of the following problems with your breasts or with breastfeeding your baby while in the hospital? Please check (✓) all that apply.
   ☐ Attachment difficulties   ☐ Sleepy baby   ☐ Preference for one breast
   ☐ Engorgement   ☐ Sore nipples   ☐ Not enough milk
   ☐ None   ☐ Other:_____

17. While in the hospital, was your baby given any supplements?   ☐ Yes   ☐ No
   If yes, please check (✓) all that apply.
   ☐ Formula   ☐ Water (plain)   ☐ Sugar water
   How were supplements given?   ☐ Bottle   ☐ Syringe   ☐ Dropper   ☐ Other:_____

18. While in the hospital, was your baby given a pacifier?   ☐ Yes   ☐ No

19. Did you and your baby go home at the same time?   ☐ Yes   ☐ No

20. How old was the baby at discharge?_____

163

21. Are you currently having vaginal bleeding? ☐ Yes ☐ No
Have your menstrual periods returned? ☐ Yes ☐ No Date of last menstrual period:_____

22. Which of the following family planning methods are you using or do you plan to use? ☐ None
☐ Birth control pills ☐ Other:_____

FEEDING HISTORY

23. How many times in 24 hours are you currently breastfeeding your baby?
☐ Less than 8 times ☐ 8-12 times (every 2-3 hours) ☐ More than 12 times

24. What is the longest time between breastfeedings? Day:_____ Night:_____

25. How long does your baby nurse on each breast?_____

26. While nursing, do you sense any of the following in your breasts?
☐ Filling ☐ Burning ☐ Milk dripping from other breast
☐ Tingling ☐ Emptying ☐ None of the above
☐ Other_____

27. Who decides when the feeding is over? ☐ Mother ☐ Baby

28. At home, has your baby received:
☐ Water ☐ Formula ☐ Liquids, other than formula ☐ Any solids

29. How many times in 24 hours has your baby had: Wet diapers: _____ Bowel movements: _____

30. Does your baby spit up? ☐ Never ☐ Occasionally ☐ Often

31. Is the baby content or sleeping between feedings? ☐ Never ☐ Occasionally ☐ Often

32. Has your baby had any prolonged crying spells? ☐ Never ☐ Occasionally ☐ Often

33. Is your baby given a pacifier? ☐ Never ☐ Occasionally ☐ Often

34. Have you had any of the following problems with your breasts or with breastfeeding since coming home?
☐ Baby always hungry
☐ Baby prefers one breast
☐ Baby not interested
☐ Other: _____
☐ Cracked/bleeding nipples
☐ Nipple pain
☐ Breast pain
☐ Painfully full breast(s)
☐ Not enough milk
☐ None of the above

35. Have you used any of the following? Please check (✓) all that apply.
☐ Hand expression
☐ Breast pump
☐ Breast cream
☐ Nursing bra (no underwire)
☐ Nursing bra (with underwire)
☐ Breast or nipple shield
☐ None of the above
☐ Other: _____

36. Your bra size: before pregnancy _____ now _____

FAMILY HISTORY

37. Does anyone on either side of the baby's family have any of the following?

☐ Allergy (food)
☐ Allergy (asthma)
☐ Allergy (eczema)
☐ Other:

☐ Allergy (hay fever)
☐ Cancer (breast)
☐ Diabetes

☐ Genetic disease
☐ Thyroid disease
☐ None of the above

38. How are members of your family adjusting to the new baby?
☐ Very well   ☐ Reasonably well   ☐ Poorly   ☐ Very poorly

39. Was your baby planned?   ☐ Yes   ☐ No

40. When did you decide to breastfeed this baby?
☐ Before pregnancy   ☐ During pregnancy   ☐ After delivery

41. How did you prepare for breastfeeding?
☐ Classes   ☐ Reading   ☐ Other:

42. Were you breastfed?   ☐ Yes   ☐ No   ☐ Not known

43. Was your baby's father breastfed?   ☐ Yes   ☐ No   ☐ Not known

44. How many previous babies have you breastfed? _____
    How long? _____ Why did you stop? _____

45. Why do you wish to breastfeed your baby? _____

46. Is there anyone in your household/family who feels you should not breastfeed this baby? ☐ Yes ☐ No

47. For how long do you plan to breastfeed this baby? _____

48. Why do you think you will discontinue breastfeeding at that time? _____

49. What was the highest grade or year of regular school you have completed?
    ☐ Less than 6 years   ☐ High school (12 years)   ☐ 4-year college (16 years)
    ☐ Elementary school (6 years)   ☐ 2-year college (14 years)   ☐ Graduate school (17+ years)
    ☐ Junior high school (9 years)

50. Usual occupation? Mother: _____ Father: _____
    When does mother plan to return to work? _____

NUTRITION

51. Did you see a nutritionist during your pregnancy? ☐ Yes ☐ No

52. Are there any foods that you avoid eating? ☐ Yes ☐ No If yes, what:
Why?_____

53. Are you now on any of these special diets?
☐ High protein ☐ Low salt ☐ Diabetic
☐ Low fat ☐ Weight loss ☐ No special diet
☐ Other:_____
If yes, who suggested the diet?_____

54. Are you trying to lose weight at this time? ☐ Yes ☐ No If yes, how much?_____
How? ☐ Less food/more exercise ☐ Program:_____ ☐ Other:_____

55. Are you a vegetarian? ☐ Yes ☐ No
If yes, do you consume: ☐ Milk products (milk, cheese, yogurt) ☐ Eggs?

56. How would you rate your appetite presently? ☐ Good ☐ Fair ☐ Poor

57. How would you describe the type and amount of food in your household?
☐ Enough of the kind you want
☐ Enough, but not always the kind you want
☐ Sometimes not enough
☐ Often not enough

168

58. Are you receiving any of the following?
   ☐ Food stamps   ☐ Medi-Cal   ☐ Donated food/meals
   ☐ WIC   ☐ AFDC/welfare   ☐ None of the above
   ☐ Other:_____

59. Do you have someone to help you shop and prepare meals?   ☐ Yes   ☐ No

60. How many times a day do you eat meals:_____ and snacks:_____

61. How many cups (8 oz.) of the following liquids do you usually drink per day?
   _____ Water   _____ Sodas with sugar   _____ Coffee
   _____ Juice   _____ Diet soda, diet punch   _____ Tea
   _____ Milk   _____ Punch, Kool-Aid, Tang   _____ Other:_____

LIFESTYLE
62. How often are you now drinking beer, wine, hard liquor, or mixed drinks?
   ☐ Daily   ☐ Weekly   ☐ Monthly   ☐ Never
   When you drink, how many drinks do you have?   ☐ One   ☐ Two   ☐ Three   ☐ More

63. How many cigarettes do you smoke each day?
   ☐ Do not smoke   ☐ Fewer than 10 cigarettes   ☐ 11-20 cigarettes   ☐ More than 20 cigarettes

169

64. How often are you currently exercising (besides housework, child care)? _____
    What types of exercise do you do? _____

65. Do you feel you are getting adequate rest? ☐ Never ☐ Occasionally ☐ Often

66. Having a new baby can be a stressful time for the family. What other stresses are present in your home?
    ☐ Relationship difficulties
    ☐ Lack of help with home/child care
    ☐ Moving
    ☐ Financial concerns
    ☐ Drug or alcohol use
    ☐ Illness/death in the family
    ☐ Other: _____
    ☐ None of the above

67. Who lives with you in your home? _____

68. Do you have any other concerns about yourself, your baby, or your family's health that you would like to discuss during your appointment? ☐ Yes ☐ No
    If yes, what? _____

MATERNAL ANTHROPOMETRY

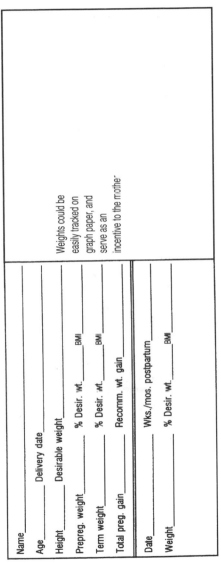

Name _____

Age _____ Delivery date _____

Height _____ Desirable weight _____

Prepreg. weight _____ % Desir. wt. _____ BMI _____

Term weight _____ % Desir. wt. _____ BMI _____

Total preg. gain _____ Recomm. wt. gain _____

Date _____ Wks./mos. postpartum _____

Weight _____ % Desir. wt. _____ BMI _____

Weights could be easily tracked on graph paper, and serve as an incentive to the mother.

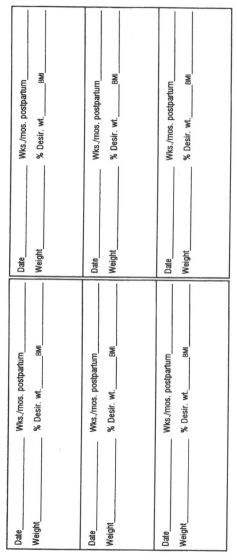

Date _____ Wks./mos. postpartum _____

Weight _____ % Desir. wt. _____ BMI _____

Date _____ Wks./mos. postpartum _____

Weight _____ % Desir. wt. _____ BMI _____

Date _____ Wks./mos. postpartum _____

Weight _____ % Desir. wt. _____ BMI _____

Date _____ Wks./mos. postpartum _____

Weight _____ % Desir. wt. _____ BMI _____

Date _____ Wks./mos. postpartum _____

Weight _____ % Desir. wt. _____ BMI _____

Date _____ Wks./mos. postpartum _____

Weight _____ % Desir. wt. _____ BMI _____

MOTHER'S PHYSICAL EXAM

	Height	Prepreg. wt.	Term wt.	Current wt.	Temperature	Blood Pressure
Postpartum days/weeks						
General Appearance			Thyroid			
BREASTS	RIGHT				LEFT	
AREOLA						
NIPPLES						
SECRETION						
OTHER						

INFANT'S PHYSICAL EXAM

DATE	AGE	WEIGHT (pounds)	(kg.)	HEIGHT (inches)	(cm.)	H.C. (inches)	(cm.)
	Birth						
Discharge:							
Today:							

GENERAL/BEHAVIOR

Temp.

Head	Heart
Eyes	Pulses
Ears	Abdomen
Nose	Genitalia
Mouth	Extremities
Thorax	Neuro
Lungs	Skin

174

ORAL-MOTOR EXAMINATION/FUNCTION

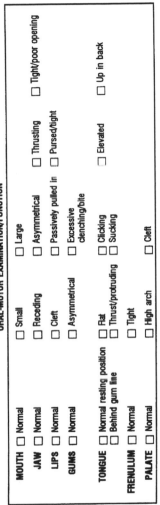

MOUTH ☐ Normal ☐ Small ☐ Large

JAW ☐ Normal ☐ Receding ☐ Asymmetrical ☐ Thrusting ☐ Tight/poor opening

LIPS ☐ Normal ☐ Cleft ☐ Passively pulled in ☐ Pursed/tight

GUMS ☐ Normal ☐ Asymmetrical ☐ Excessive clenching/bite

TONGUE ☐ Normal resting position ☐ Flat ☐ Clicking ☐ Elevated ☐ Up in back
☐ Behind gum line ☐ Thrust/protruding ☐ Sucking

FRENULUM ☐ Normal ☐ Tight

PALATE ☐ Normal ☐ High arch ☐ Cleft

175

BREASTFEEDING OBSERVATION

Position used:
- [ ] Cradle
- [ ] Side-sitting
- [ ] Other:_____

Infant interest:
- [ ] Hungry, eager, goes easily to breast
- [ ] Willing but not insistent
- [ ] Willing but distractable
- [ ] Willing, falls asleep quickly
- [ ] Sleepy, totally disinterested
- [ ] Awake, will not attach
- [ ] Awake, hungry, vigorously refuses

Rooting:
- [ ] Normal
- [ ] Frantic, disorganized
- [ ] Depressed/absent
- [ ] Tongue back/flat

Attachment:
- [ ] Adequate
- [ ] Drops back
- [ ] Tongue malposition
- [ ] Lips retracted
- [ ] Arches
- [ ] Cries
- [ ] Refuses
- [ ] Other:_____

Milk ejection reflex:
- [ ] Prior to attachment
- [ ] Hyperactive
- [ ] After attachment, _____ sec / min
- [ ] Not apparent after _____ sec / min

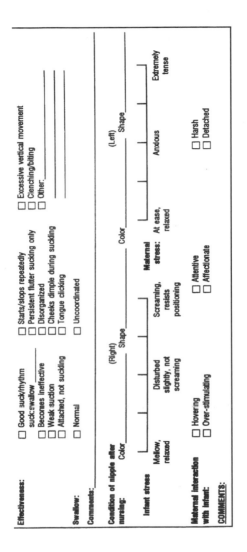

Effectiveness:
- ☐ Good suck/rhythm suck:swallow
- ☐ Becomes ineffective
- ☐ Weak suction
- ☐ Attached, not suckling
- ☐ Starts/stops repeatedly
- ☐ Persistent flutter sucking only
- ☐ Disorganized
- ☐ Cheeks dimple during suckling
- ☐ Tongue clicking
- ☐ Excessive vertical movement
- ☐ Clenching/biting
- ☐ Other:_____

Swallow: ☐ Normal ☐ Uncoordinated

Comments:

Condition of nipple after nursing:
(Right) Color_____ Shape_____
(Left) Color_____ Shape_____

Infant stress:
Mellow, relaxed — Disturbed slightly, not screaming — Screaming, resists positioning

Maternal stress:
At ease, relaxed — Anxious — Extremely tense

Maternal interaction with infant:
- ☐ Hovering
- ☐ Over-stimulating
- ☐ Attentive
- ☐ Affectionate
- ☐ Harsh
- ☐ Detached

COMMENTS:

Appendix I

Conversion Tables

TABLE I-1. CONVERSION OF POUNDS TO KILOGRAMS FOR PEDIATRIC WEIGHTS

POUNDS →	0	1	2	3	4	5	6	7	8	9
0	0.00	0.45	0.90	1.36	1.81	2.26	2.72	3.17	3.62	4.08
10	4.53	4.98	5.44	5.89	6.35	6.80	7.25	7.71	8.16	8.61
20	9.07	9.52	9.97	10.43	10.88	11.34	11.79	12.24	12.70	13.15
30	13.60	14.06	14.51	14.96	15.42	15.87	16.32	16.78	17.23	17.69
40	18.14	18.59	19.05	19.50	19.95	20.41	20.86	21.31	21.77	22.22
50	22.68	23.13	23.58	24.04	24.49	24.94	25.40	25.85	26.30	26.76
60	27.21	27.66	28.12	28.57	29.03	29.48	29.93	30.39	30.84	31.29
70	31.75	32.20	32.65	33.11	33.56	34.02	34.47	34.92	35.38	35.83
80	36.28	36.74	37.19	37.64	38.10	38.55	39.00	39.46	39.91	40.37
90	40.82	41.27	41.73	42.18	42.63	43.09	43.54	43.99	44.45	44.90

100	45.36	45.81	46.26	46.72	47.17	47.62	48.08	48.53	48.98	49.44
110	49.89	50.34	50.80	51.25	51.71	52.16	52.61	53.07	53.52	53.97
120	54.43	54.88	55.33	55.79	56.24	56.70	57.15	57.60	58.06	58.51
130	58.96	59.42	59.87	60.32	60.78	61.23	61.68	62.14	62.59	63.05
140	63.50	63.95	64.41	64.86	65.31	65.77	66.22	66.67	67.13	67.58
150	68.04	68.49	68.94	69.40	69.85	70.30	70.76	71.21	71.66	72.12
160	72.57	73.02	73.48	73.93	74.39	74.84	75.29	75.75	76.20	76.65
170	77.11	77.56	78.01	78.47	78.92	79.38	79.83	80.82	80.74	81.19
180	81.64	82.10	82.55	83.00	83.46	83.91	84.36	84.82	85.27	85.73
190	86.18	86.68	87.09	87.54	87.99	88.45	88.90	89.35	89.81	90.26
200	90.72	91.17	91.62	92.08	92.53	92.98	93.44	93.89	94.34	94.80

TABLE I-2. CONVERSION OF POUNDS AND OUNCES TO KILOGRAMS FOR PEDIATRIC WEIGHTS

Pounds	Kilograms	Ounces	Kilograms
1	0.454	1	0.028
2	0.907	2	0.057
3	1.361	3	0.085
4	1.814	4	0.113
5	2.268	5	0.142
6	2.722	6	0.170
7	3.175	7	0.198
8	3.629	8	0.227
9	4.082	9	0.255
10	4.536	10	0.283
11	4.990	11	0.312
12	5.443	12	0.340
13	5.897	13	0.369
		14	0.397
		15	0.425

Appendix J

Standardized Height and Weight Growth Charts

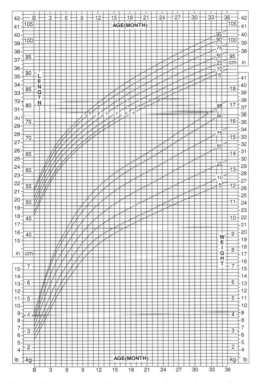

Boys: Birth to age 36 months–physical growth (length, weight). NCHS percentiles
Source: Charts on pp. 181–182 are modified from PVV Hamill et al: Physical growth: National Center for Health Statistics percentiles. Am J Clin Nutr 32: 607–29, 1979. Data from the Fels Research Institute, Wright State University School of Medicine, Yellow Springs, OH.

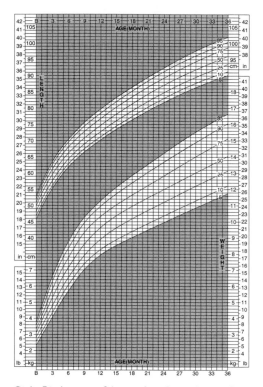

Girls: Birth to age 36 months–physical growth (length, weight). NCHS percentiles